D0227622

Rehabilitation for Work Matters

Rehabilitation for Work Matters

Jim Ford, Gordon Parker, Fiona Ford, Diana Kloss,
Simon Pickvance and Philip Sawney

Foreword by
Professor Dame Carol Black
National Director for Health and Work

Radcliffe Publishing
Oxford • New York

Radcliffe Publishing Ltd
18 Marcham Road
Abingdon
Oxon OX14 1AA
United Kingdom

www.radcliffe-oxford.com
Electronic catalogue and worldwide online ordering facility.

British Library Cataloguing in Publication Data

A catalogue record for this book is available from the British Library.

ISBN-13: 978 185775 786 6

Typeset by Pindar New Zealand (Egan Reid), Auckland, New Zealand
Printed and bound by Hobbs the Printers Ltd, Southampton, Hampshire, UK

Contents

To the (late) Marie Ford and to Mary Ford, who inspired and continue to inspire hope in disability employment.

Foreword

For a long time physicians have known about occupational disease – that is, the familiar hazards of particular kinds of work. However, against this we have been less aware of the hazards of not working and the consequences of worklessness, whether in fit people or in people with illnesses or disabilities that should not deny them opportunities to work.

It has become only too evident that ceasing to work – in the right work – is a source of another disorder, namely a decline in general health and well-being. It is one that we might call non-occupational disease, with all the problems which that state can bring. Often worklessness, legitimised by sickness certification, results in permanent withdrawal from working life, frequently marked by formal retirement on the grounds of ill health.

Among our concerns as practitioners should be the crucial interplay between work and health and well-being. None should need reminding of the importance of work to personal and family well-being, and to dignity, self-esteem and sense of purpose, with recognition of the essential social function of work.

Clinicians emphasise the importance of rest, and therefore of relief from work, to aid the natural healing that occurs with the passage of time. However, that understanding is often unmatched by advice and encouragement about timely return to work following illness or injury, and the benefits of this for health and well-being.

This is the reason for this volume. It is designed to fill a gap that is common in clinical practice, by showing ways of helping and encouraging patients to return to or even to remain in work when they fall sick or are injured or disabled. It is heavily based on the personal experience of the authors, and is illustrated by vignettes that highlight significant clinical dilemmas.

Even if it is not true that 'hard work never killed anyone', it was a physician, no less than Galen of Pergamon who, in AD 172, described work as 'nature's best physician and as essential to human happiness.' The following chapters offer practitioners from primary and secondary care ways in which to test Galen's prescription.

Professor Dame Carol Black
National Director for Health and Work
March 2008

Preface

Happy, healthy and here.

Occupational health professionals often describe their role as keeping working people 'happy, healthy and here.' Within this description, the specialisation can be said to have two components, namely minimising the adverse effects of work on health, and mitigating the effects of *ill* health on work. This book complements the earlier volume, *Occupational Health Matters in General Practice*, but concentrates on keeping people 'here' – which is mostly about mitigating the effects of ill health on their work. However, it is impossible to neatly dissect out and disentangle rather trite statements like this. For in returning vulnerable people to work we risk the adverse effects of work impinging on their health, and we may encourage inappropriate attendance when unfit, or *presenteeism*.

Therefore this book has been written as a general support for healthcare professionals who want to help their patients to remain actively in employment. It is not intended to be a textbook of occupational medicine, nor is it aimed at occupational health professionals, although such practitioners will find it a useful source of tips and practical information. Neither is it a highly scientific work. Rather it is a practical guide aimed at practitioners, especially in primary care, who are tasked with a number of responsibilities (including certification) which are complementary to workplace health, and who may have very little interest in these, or may even find them irksome. It is anticipated that lay rehabilitationists, professionals allied to medicine and specialists in other fields may also find it a useful support in keeping their patients of working age economically active and healthy.

The bulk of the text has been written by two occupational health consultants, one of whom has focused on economic inactivity while the other has focused on fitness for work. Two chapters have been written by primary care workers – one by a GP with a special interest in economic inactivity, and the other from the perspective of a lay occupational health adviser. Finally, specialist chapters have been written by experts in social security and occupational health law. There is some overlap between chapters, which is designed to encourage reflection and to demonstrate crossover between different practitioners and approaches.

The complex nature of the relationships and drivers is illustrated by a series of clinical vignettes written by the authors or their distinguished colleagues that should prove valuable as case discussions or clinical scenarios for use in problem-based learning.

Jim Ford
March 2008

About the authors

Dr Jim Ford MSc, MFOM, DDAM, DRCOG, certMHS, FAMS
Consultant Occupational Health Physician, University Hospital Aintree and Salus Occupational Health & Safety; Honorary Lecturer, School of Health and Postgraduate Medicine, University of Central Lancashire, Preston
Jim's interest in employment was kindled while he was working in a labour exchange as an undergraduate. A dozen years in general practice led him to the medical civil service, where he discovered the clinical, social, psychological and epidemiological phenomenon of health-related economic inactivity. A spell in primary care policy at the Department of Health led to his becoming Medical Director of the Job Retention and Rehabilitation Pilots, before returning to clinical practice in the shipbuilding, nuclear and munitions industries with WellWork. Since 2005, he has worked in local government for Salus, and more recently also for University Hospital Aintree. He has published on the subject of incapacity, and was the professional adviser to Smoke-Free Liverpool, the persistence of which ultimately achieved a workplace smoking ban in England, which he regards as his greatest professional achievement to date.

Dr Fiona Ford MBE, MRCGP
Senior Lecturer in General Practice, Lancashire School of Health and Postgraduate Medicine, University of Central Lancashire, Preston
Fiona has been a practising GP for more than 25 years, and has been researching incapacity and sickness certification for over 10 years. She was awarded an MBE in 2007 for her work on developing and evaluating the Condition Management Programmes to help claimants of incapacity benefits to manage their long-term conditions in order to return to work. She is on the National Institute for Clinical Excellence expert panel, working on guidelines for long-term sickness and incapacity. She also has special interests in healthcare for

ethnic-minority populations and in medical education, having worked on the development of the new community-oriented undergraduate medical curriculum at the University of Liverpool.

Diana Kloss LLB LLM, Hon FFOM
Barrister and Honorary Senior Lecturer, Department of Occupational and Environmental Medicine, University of Manchester; Chairman of Employment Tribunals
Diana was an academic lawyer at the School of Law of the University of Manchester until her retirement in 2002. She retains her connection with the University as an Honorary Senior Lecturer in Occupational Health Law. In 1986 she was called to the Bar, and she practises from St John's Buildings in Manchester, specialising in employment law. In 1995 she was appointed part-time Chairman of Employment Tribunals in Manchester and Liverpool.

Diana is the author of a number of books and papers, principally *Occupational Health Law* (published by Blackwell Science, Oxford, in 2005), which is now in its fourth edition. She lectures to occupational health professionals throughout the UK, and writes a regular column in the journal Occupational Health at Work. She has been elected an Honorary Fellow of the Faculty of Occupational Medicine of the Royal College of Physicians.

She is also a former member of the Expert Advisory Group on AIDS and the UK Advisory Panel for Health Care Workers Infected with Blood-borne Viruses, and a member of the CJD Incidents Panel and the Industrial Injuries Advisory Council.

Dr Gordon Parker MA, FRCP, FFOM, MRCGP, CMIOSH
Consultant in Occupational Medicine, Lancashire Teaching Hospitals NHS Foundation Trust; Honorary Clinical Lecturer, University of Manchester; Group Medical Adviser to the Ranks Hovis McDougall group
After five years as a principal in general practice in Morecambe, Gordon trained in occupational medicine in the power generation industry. He subsequently served as University Occupational Physician and Head of Health and Safety Services at the University of Manchester, and then as Group Medical Adviser to the Rank Hovis McDougall group of food companies, before taking up his present post of Consultant in Occupational Medicine at Lancashire Teaching Hospitals NHS Foundation Trust in Preston.

He has a continuing interest in the interface between primary care and occupational medicine, and has published work on training in occupational medicine for GPs.

He is a former Regional Adviser and Training Dean for the Faculty of Occupational Medicine, and an Honorary Clinical Lecturer at the University of Manchester.

Simon Pickvance
Senior Adviser, Sheffield Occupational Health Advisory Service; Honorary Research Fellow, School for Health and Related Research, University of Sheffield
Simon has a particular interest in health and safety in the metal industries, occupational stress, and the burden of work-related ill health. His previous publications include *Health and Safety in the Steel Industry* (published by IMF, Geneva, in 1999) and the *Manual of Occupational Health in Primary Care* (published by Sheffield Occupational Health Advisory Service, Sheffield, in 2003).

Dr Philip Sawney BSc, MB BS, MBA, MRCGP, DDAM, DOcc Med, DGM, DRCOG
Deputy Chief Medical Adviser (retired), Department for Work and Pensions, UK
Philip has worked as a principal in general practice, occupational medicine and disability assessment medicine. He has also worked as a consultant for the UK Know How Fund in Bulgaria and Estonia. He was a GP Tutor in south-west London and, more recently, an examiner for the Faculty of Occupational Medicine.

Acknowledgements

The authors are most grateful to Dr Charles Vivian for reading through the manuscript and for his perceptive comments. We are also grateful to Professor Mansel Aylward CB, Professor David Haslam PRCGP and John Ballard for contributing their clinical anecdotes which add much colour to the points made in the text.

CHAPTER 1

Introduction

SICKNESS CERTIFICATION: A GOOD PLACE TO START?

Certification of sickness for employers is a task which has been the responsibility of GPs for nearly a century, and is the one aspect of their work relating to workplace health that they cannot avoid. There is no indication that it is a task which is likely to be removed. Rather, if anything, we might expect the clinical governance process which has improved the rest of primary care to spread into this area. It must thus be judged as a core task in primary care, so this is a good place to begin a book about rehabilitation and return to work, so that the wider potential for health improvement which the invitation to participate positively in the certification process offers can be explored. Chapter 4 will examine certification in greater depth. The rest of this chapter will consider what we actually mean by the words used in this field.

What is certification?

Sickness certification fulfils a number of roles in working-age society. It provides a universal structure which forces an employee who feels unfit to attend their primary care practitioner at around the time when a simple illness should be resolving. It also provides a form of attestation that the person is too ill to attend work, which enables an employer to accept that the employee is physically or mentally unable to work. Some employers might judge that, in requiring the effort to attend a GP, it also disincentives absence. However, other employers feel that GP certificates legitimise trivial causes of absence. The fact that certification results in a paper transaction between employer, employee and GP is often forgotten, for this creates opportunities for further communication that are rarely exploited, but which will be explored in this book.

Duty of certification

Many GPs nonetheless remain deeply uneasy about the task of certification, and complain that it introduces role conflict into their duty as patient advocates. However, good patient advocacy surely requires that patients are made fully aware of the possible long-term health outcomes of their behaviour. Patients who may be struggling with the effects on their working ability of a new medical condition, such as diabetes, or with new working practices, such as being located in a call centre, may be desperate for the respite of a couple of weeks 'on the sick.' But will things be any different when they return after this time? Probably not, and on return there may be some considerable catching up to do, if only with the office politics. Inevitably, there will be a temptation to ask for another note, and then another, and who can blame a GP for giving a longer duration?

'Diagnoses' on sick notes

It is often clear that the diagnosis which is written on a certificate has little to do with what is actually happening to the employee. One of the most difficult areas concerns the need for a person to stay off sick because they are 'required at home' to provide support for a partner with a serious illness or for a handicapped child. Individuals who enjoy generous sick pay may be tempted to send in a sick note when they should really be requesting (unpaid) compassionate leave. However, their employer is not funded to cover such lengthy absences; the consequential costs will be carried by the whole organisation, but in practice the burden of replacing their duties will fall on their colleagues. And when they do return to work, they may not be surprised to witness one of their colleagues subsequently producing a sick note for 'stress'! In the longer term, such absence will affect the efficiency of their unit, and might lead to outsourcing to an external private provider who is unlikely to accept such practice.

THE COST OF ABSENCE

We are frequently reminded of the cost of sickness absence to employers: £13.4 billion a year in salaries alone, according to the CBI. But the greatest burden is not on the employer but on the colleagues of the absent employee, or indeed on the individual returning from sickness.

When businesses claim they are losing huge sums through sickness absence, it assumes that productivity would be dramatically improved if all workers attended 100% of their contracted hours. The reality in most situations, however, is that other workers pick up the work from absent colleagues, frequently through unpaid overtime and lost breaks. One survey of UK workers found that two-thirds stay late at least once a week, half take work home and two-fifths have to work at weekends at least some of the time – simply because of the demands placed on them. Organisations have been trimmed over recent years to achieve maximum output from the smallest number of employees, but because jobs are not designed to allow for sickness absence, most short-term labour shortages are absorbed not by the employer's purse but by an already stretched workforce. And the consequences of this extra workload: longer hours, greater pressure and increased demands on workers already at elevated risk to their health from work-related stress.

For some people, however, being absent means work piling up unattended. Many people will have experienced the post-holiday dread: countless emails, letters, voicemails and tasks with urgent deadlines. Sadly, many people off sick for prolonged periods will have that very same feeling – nothing has been done to ease their workload in their absence. If the cause of their sickness in the first place was work-related stress, what better way to hamper their return?

John Ballard

John Ballard is director of the At Work Partnership and editor of the journal *Occupational Health [at Work]*.

Duration of sick notes

It is tempting for a busy GP, when faced with repeated requests for sick notes from a patient whom they are expecting to be recovering, to issue a certificate of long duration such as 8 or 13 weeks or even 'ufn' (until further notice). However, government statistics suggest that many long absentees fail to return to work altogether. Providing shorter certificates enables regular reviews and creates opportunities for encouraging the person to return to meaningful activity, as a prelude to work. Such investment by the GP may be wearing and repetitive, but allowing the patient to lapse into economic inactivity will gift them plenty of time and opportunity to make many appointments in future!

Health risks of unemployment

Research suggests that being workless incurs a risk to health equivalent to smoking 200 cigarettes per day. Health risks and life expectancy are worse than those for many killer diseases, and there are greater risks attached to worklessness than to most dangerous jobs, even those in construction or the North Sea. In particular, the general suicide rate is increased sixfold in the longer-term unemployed, and in young men who have been unemployed for just 6 months it is increased 40-fold.

Economic inactivity and poverty

Spending the rest of one's working life on benefits inevitably leads to lower prosperity, and possibly also poverty and ill health. Equally, although a 'full' early pension, without actuarial reduction and with extra years granted for ill health, may seem alluring for the declining number of employees who are still entitled to a defined benefit pension, it may be too late before the person realises that, at best, this actually means half-pay for the remainder of their life, with no increases due to promotion or seniority and further growth determined by the stock market or the retail price index!

WHAT IS REHABILITATION FOR WORK?

Rehabilitation for work is rehabilitation that is orientated towards the goal of achieving gainful occupation and economic independence in an impaired, ill, injured or disabled person of working age. It is a modern evolution of vocational rehabilitation, with a stronger emphasis on achieving sustainable employment in the *open labour market* as the ultimate goal. Traditional vocational rehabilitation was developed with ex-servicemen after the Second World War, and continued up to the 1970s using a medical model for rehabilitation, with sheltered workshops and other placements outside the open market for employment.

Nowadays, sheltered workshops are exceptional, and even quite severely disabled people work in mainstream jobs with support and encouragement. The fighter pilot, Douglas Bader, is legendary in this context. After losing both of his legs in action he returned to flying Spitfires, and when he was captured, his captors had to remove his artificial legs to prevent his repeated attempts to escape. In modern times the Cambridge physicist, Professor Stephen Hawking, continues to achieve international acclaim as a physicist despite severe disablement with motor neuron disease. For anybody studying successful adaptation to disability, Professor Hawking's personal website (www.hawking.org.uk) is worth more than a passing glance to see what it feels like to have a successful career with a profound disability.

Although return to paid work remains the ultimate goal, there are a number of intermediate stops along the way, such as training and voluntary work. The word 'rehabilitation' implies an active process of recovery to a previous state. However, the same word is commonly also applied to people who are not recovering, but who instead are trying to overcome the disabling effects of an inherited condition resulting in impairment, such as learning disability or spina bifida.

There are two other useful definitions of rehabilitation used in this field which illustrate the wider stakeholders. A joint working group of the Trades Union Congress and the Association of British Insurers set out that 'Rehabilitation should restore a person who has been injured or suffered an illness to as productive and as independent a lifestyle as possible through the use of medical, functional and vocational interventions.' The British Society of Rehabilitation Medicine describes rehabilitation as 'A process of active change by which a person who has become disabled acquires the knowledge and skills needed for optimal physical, psychological and social function.'

WHAT IS DISABILITY?

Disability means difficulties encountered by an individual when performing particular functions. These may be physical and/or mental impairments. It implies nothing about causation or diagnosis, but is concerned with the limitation of activities and restriction of participation in people with physical and/or mental conditions or impairments – that is, it is an entirely *functional* concept. Disabled people often prefer to describe their disability not in medical language, but in terms which reflect the extent to which the outside world has adapted to their needs. This is described as the social model of disability.

WHAT IS IMPAIRMENT?

Impairment is the underlying change in the mind or body, which causes the disability. For example, difficulty in getting about might be caused by a hemiplegia, perhaps due to a stroke or a brain injury. An impairment is usually described in *medical* terms, and can be caused by an underlying medical condition or an injury. It is thus a significant, demonstrable deviation or loss of body structure or function, sometimes referred to as 'loss of faculty.'

WHAT IS INCAPACITY?

Incapacity means a lack of capability of an individual to undertake a set of tasks which would be considered normal for a person of their age or background. For example, a person who is suffering from a mental health condition may lack sufficient mental capacity to sign documents. In the context of rehabilitation for work, when we talk about incapacity, we normally mean incapacity for work – that is, reduced capacity for and functioning at work (i.e. for participating in economically gainful activity). It can be difficult to distinguish between 'capacity' and 'performance' where the latter also depends on motivation and effort, which therefore complicates the assessment of incapacity, as we shall see later.

WHY THESE TERMS MATTER: OBJECTIVITY AND SUBJECTIVITY

In the past, these terms have been used quite loosely, and even interchangeably. However, the modern understanding about different models of disability and the context of assessment means that we need to treat the terms more precisely, especially as medical decisions often result in resource consequences elsewhere. For this reason they are defined in UK law for Social Security terms. The summary table which follows is repeated again in Chapter 9. Note that the terms 'disease', 'impairment' and 'injury' are *objective*, implying that impartial evidence exists to support their existence. By contrast, 'illness' and 'disability' are *subjective* concepts which may vary from person to person. Both subjective and objective factors will influence the outcome of incapacity or sickness in an individual.

THE DISTINCTION BETWEEN KEY TERMS

Disease is objective, medically diagnosed pathology (i.e. it is a disorder of structure or function of the human organism).

Impairment is significant, demonstrable deviation or loss of body structure or function, sometimes referred to as 'loss of faculty.'

Symptoms are bodily or mental sensations that reach consciousness (e.g. aches, pains, fatigue, breathlessness, anxiety).

Illness is the subjective feeling of being unwell (i.e. it is an internal, personal experience).

Disability is the limitation of activities and restriction of participation in people with physical and/or mental conditions or impairments.

Sickness, or *the sick role*, is a social status accorded to the ill person by society, with exemption from normal social roles and carrying specific rights and responsibilities (i.e. it is an external, social phenomenon).

Incapacity is reduced capacity for and functioning at work. It is difficult to distinguish between 'capacity' and 'performance' where the latter also depends on motivation and effort.

THE BIOMEDICAL MODEL

As physicians we are very familiar with the biomedical model, namely the presentation of symptoms, and diagnosis by history-taking examination and investigations, leading to commencement of treatment and recovery. However, we observe that despite scientific rigour, not everyone gets better, and symptoms may be misleading, especially when they are subjective and the absence of objective investigations and signs does not mean that there is no underlying impairment – it may just be that it has not been diagnosed yet. The Cartesian model of pain as a manifestation of underlying disorder similarly ignores the enduring effect of pain once the cause has been determined to be less than serious.

COMMON HEALTH CONDITIONS AND WORK

Common health conditions, such as ischaemic heart disease, high blood pressure, diabetes, anxiety/depression, chronic low back pain and other musculoskeletal conditions, are inexorably increasing in prevalence as the UK population ages. Indeed, public health programmes in the NHS (such as the Quality and Outcomes Framework in General Practice) are often seeking to identify these conditions early so that preventative interventions can be implemented. It would be unfortunate if such interventions led to patients 'hanging up their boots' prematurely and suffering the health consequences of economic inactivity, simply because they had been made aware of asymptomatic conditions such as high blood pressure.

The effect of common health conditions on work

None of these common health conditions necessarily permanently prevent an individual from working (although they may do so temporarily), but they may make some of the *demands* of work more difficult, and it may be especially difficult to cope if, at the same time, the individual's or employer's economic circumstances are driving up expectations. In addition, changes in the workplace, perhaps driven by external economic circumstances such as globalisation, can make it seem less supportive, or even hostile.

The individual may *lose their confidence* at work and begin to feel that they can no longer continue with their usual occupation. In the absence of good occupational health or vocational support, they may see no alternative but to seek sickness certification or even ill health retirement, citing the common health condition which they may have been diagnosed with and lived with for several years. However, there are actually quite a number of interventions (as will be discussed later in this volume) which can be put in place to enable the employee to continue in their own or another job. Later on we shall also explore how legislation against discrimination due to age and disability can assist by preventing discrimination in employment and providing a structure within which an employee or his adviser can increase the likelihood of a successful or sustained return to work.

THE IMPACT OF INJURY

Dr Stephen Duckworth, a doctor who is Chief Executive of an organisation called Disability Matters, acquired a spinal injury while he was a medical student. In his lectures he describes the 'psychology of change' which follows catastrophic injury as being rather similar to the grieving reaction of bereavement. Initially there is shock and disbelief, which is followed by despair as the reality of the permanent state of relative dependence and limitation dawns and the person sinks deeper into a state of depression, which can last for weeks, months or even years.

Psychological adaptation

After some weeks or months, perhaps encouraged by a partial physical or mental recovery, the disabled person begins to see some positive opportunities, and they enter a period of experimentation and even optimism as they discover new ways of doing familiar tasks. Unfortunately, as with non-disabled individuals, there are some disabled people who are naturally pessimistic, or who have over-zealous carers, and who therefore cannot easily reach this stage. An observant primary care practitioner may spot such cases and encourage the disabled person and their carer to allow sensible experimentation, and not to see disablement as a 'life sentence' for both of them.

Adverse effect of assessment on recovery

An unfortunate consequence of acquired disability which has been identified by the psychology of change model is that economic and social factors can get in the way of recovery. For example, a person who is just discovering new ways to get about or who is learning to cope with a disfiguring injury may need to be assessed at a medical centre in a neighbouring town, perhaps during the rush hour. When they attend, inevitably the history and examination which are undertaken will highlight what they *cannot* do, and the whole process can be humiliating and demoralising. If benefits are reduced as a result, the adverse impact may be heightened, even though this in fact represents the recognition of strong recovery. However, it is not easy for an impaired and disabled person to see it like that!

The effect of causation

The rate of recovery from an injury or poisoning may also be influenced by the feelings of the disabled person about the causation of the impairment. For example, if the injury occurred at work, or was due to exposure to a harmful substance, they may believe that their employer owes them a special duty of accommodation – or even greater tolerance of lengthy absence. The employer (or his insurer or solicitor) may not share this view!

OVERADAPTATION AND PRESENTEEISM

There are other disabled people whose optimism goes into overdrive, and who behave as if they are pretending that their disability does not exist. Many would regard the late Hollywood actor Christopher Reeve (who played the part of Superman) as a member of this category. Despite a severe quadriplegic neck injury, the actor was determined to walk independently. Again, the family doctor or practice nurse, with previous knowledge of the patient and their family, is well placed to use their advocacy skills to encourage the patient and his or her carers to be more realistic.

THE IMPACT OF POISONING

Poisoning is due to the ingestion, inhalation or absorption of noxious substances. Traditional workplace hazards include lead, asbestos and ionising radiation. However, occasionally some substances have been quite unexpectedly found to be toxic. For example, vinyl chloride monomer (VCM) – a gas used in the polymerisation of PVC (polyvinylchloride) – was initially considered to be benign enough to be used as an anaesthetic agent. However, it has subsequently been shown to be associated with two types of malignant liver cancer, as well as being toxic to the bones and circulation of the fingers, thus preventing affected individuals from doing some of their work tasks, as well as their hobbies, that require fine motor skills – and domestic chores such as washing dishes! Naturally, those affected will be inquisitive as to the causation, and such concerns may result in a claim against the company's insurer. The processing of such claims can take an eternity – and may stand in the way of the patient adjusting to their disability and moving on. Again, a sympathetic ear or, at other times, a measured but challenging approach from a familiar practitioner can result in the patient not allowing their unresolved concerns to prevent them from returning to their usual work, and possibly becoming unemployable.

THE IMPACT OF COMPENSATION

There are a number of systems of compensation in place in the UK, which will be discussed later on. From the point of view of recovery and return to work, the problem with all of them is the *length of time that it takes to progress to settlement*. Also, because all of these schemes are based on the principle of financial recompense for assessed loss of function, in practice they tend to incentivise slow recovery and the persistence of disablement. Perhaps the greatest danger for patients is that because of the need to demonstrate disablement at its greatest effect (but perhaps many months or even years after the event), compensation assessments by independent doctors may force the patient to underestimate their recovery or even eventually to deteriorate.

UNDERSTANDING THE 'IMPAIRMENT GAP'

Often when we see a person who is disabled for the first time, we cannot quite understand the extent of their disability compared with another person and compared with what we have measured scientifically and objectively about the underlying impairment. A good example of this is high-tone deafness. One person may experience no apparent loss in hearing ability, yet have an audiogram which looks considerably worse than that of another person who is quite markedly disabled and dependent on a hearing aid. This is because disablement itself is a *subjective* phenomenon and affects different individuals in different ways. For example, the ability to distinguish conversation against a background of noise seems to be a skill which is not usually regained once it has been lost, even with the use of modern digital hearing aids.

Similarly, one person may be more disabled by back pain than another, yet have a less 'serious' appearance on their X-rays or MRI scan (*see* page 38). Obviously this subjective response makes it difficult to be fair when disabled individuals are being assessed for compensation or for state or insurance benefits payable to those judged by an independent doctor or through a process to be incapable of work. There are many approaches to this problem, and the interested reader is referred to the textbooks on disability assessment medicine listed in the Further Reading section on page 18.

VOLITION

Variability of the subjective response within disability can give rise to a suspicion that the individual may be malingering. This subject was much debated in the nineteenth century, and has been the focus of some further interest recently. Undoubtedly, some individuals do exaggerate the effects of their disability, and may be encouraged in this by colleagues or even carers, just as there are others who minimise their symptoms to enable themselves to stay in work. More frequently, people may be unaware that they could achieve more than they feel immediately able to do, perhaps because they have not had enough or the right type of encouragement.

Body language

Careful observation of simple body language can be useful in trying to detect a patient's level of commitment to their recovery or to your assessment of it. For example, a weak handshake or the avoidance of eye contact may imply that commitment to you or their own recovery is in question. However, there is a danger in being over-reliant on such signs, as they may reflect something completely different, such as the patient's resentment about being assessed at all.

Risk of prejudice

In general, it is not helpful for the assessing practitioner to set out to challenge or trick the patient so as to prove malingering. Indeed, in so doing, the practitioner risks making him- or herself appear prejudiced. It is usually much more effective to establish the facts of a case and leave those unembellished facts to tell the tale in a report without making judgement. Tabloid newspapers are full of spectacular cases where famous or not so famous people have been captured repairing roofs or attending football matches when they are receiving compensation for injury or incapacity!

Although assessing physicians may have a definite suspicion about the possibility of malingering, they will generally serve the case best by keeping such opinions to themselves, and simply recording the facts objectively, thereby avoiding the unnecessary conflict of a direct challenge. Equally, the GP or practice nurse may have their suspicions, too, but expressing them will undermine a professional relationship that will need to continue long after the compensation/incapacity case has been closed.

Avoidance of collusion

However, this does not mean that the primary care practitioner should be tempted to collude with their patient by agreeing to something which is untrue or a blatant exaggeration. At best this will prolong the assessment process while alternative, but more objective and independent evidence is sought by other affected parties, such as the employer or insurer, and such procedures inevitably add to the bureaucratic burden of the GP. At worst, it will result in a doctor–patient relationship which is permanently dependent on the financial consequences of mutual deceit, and will be followed up by expectations of similar support in further applications for more benefits, allowances and other non-financial benefits such as re-housing, free parking and leisure passes. And if the practitioner is unfortunate enough to have 'his' patient become one of the 'scroungers' exposed by a tabloid photographer, he may find that his professional reputation is also tarnished!

ILLNESS BEHAVIOUR IN THE DISABLED PERSON AND IN OTHERS

Illness behaviour is a type of psychological response whereby we modify our behaviour according to our expectations and what we have learned. For example, older people often take to their beds when they have symptoms of a cold, or they may get up but remain in their nightclothes. Other people will move in a certain way when they have pain in their back or neck, even unknowingly making it worse by holding an ergonomically inappropriate posture. And some individuals will take up the use of aids and appliances such as walking sticks, crutches, splints, wheelchairs and 'scooters' quite inappropriately. Inspection of the ferrule of a walking stick or crutch for wear will reveal the extent to which it has actually been used to bear weight, and discrete observation of its use may show it being used on the 'wrong' side, or even just being carried or dragged. In some cases, illness behaviour becomes permanent, as it may be reinforced by partners, carers and even work colleagues who well-meaningly may prevent the disabled person from dispensing with aids or assistance.

A good place to observe illness behaviour is at a football match, especially an international one. Players will get knocked over, hobble around with what appears to be a devastating injury, and five minutes later are taking a free kick as though nothing had happened. Of course there is always a suspicion that the player might be achieving 'secondary gain', such as a penalty or the sending off of an opponent. Such suspicions may be heightened if the player is a notorious 'diver' or belongs to certain nationalities!

Handling illness behaviour in your patient

Illness behaviour is almost always instinctive and automatic, but actual consideration of volition is rarely productive in a clinical setting, as it is rarely possible to safely distinguish between instinctive and deliberate behaviour. However, a challenge will always raise the patient's guard, and may undermine a previously trusting relationship, which is an important component if the sick employee is to be supported back into work. And if you get it completely wrong, there is the risk of destroying the relationship altogether and maybe enduring the investigation of a formal complaint against you.

Slow recovery or persistent illness behaviour?

Frequently, without challenging the individual, deliberate or subconscious lack of commitment to their own recovery will sooner or later be exposed by the implementation of the treatment plan. For example, the individual may decline a course of cognitive–behavioural therapy which would help them to convert their cyclical de-motivating thoughts into positive and supportive ones, or they may decline to accept (or to implement) ergonomic or postural suggestions from their physiotherapist which would enable them to complete their recovery from a 'whiplash' injury to their neck. The experienced practitioner will be familiar with (and probably irritated by) the 'knowing' smile with which his patient dutifully informs him that yet another treatment has 'failed.' Sometimes negative responses may be reinforced by the patient's manager or carer (or on occasion even another healthcare practitioner), causing the treating practitioner to question whether the carer, manager or healthcare practitioner really does want the person to recover and return to their normal activity.

Assessment of illness and illness behaviour

Such complex human behaviour can make it difficult to evaluate exactly what is really going on with your patient. In these circumstances it is helpful to supplement the conventional medical assessment by assessing disability. A later chapter will set out a useful way of doing this by taking a detailed history of a typical day and assessing function.

THE TRAINEE NURSE WITH AN UNEXPLAINED INJURY

I was once asked to undertake a pre-employment assessment of a prospective student nurse because she had been noted at triage to be in receipt of Disability Living Allowance due to a leg injury some years before. This would normally have required her to be 'unable or virtually unable to walk', which could render her unfit to train.

However, she told me that she could now walk without any limit, and clinical examination revealed no abnormality. Furthermore, the hospital letters about the injury from many years before were unable to explain objectively the level of disability claimed by her at the time. Closer questioning revealed that she actually had a very large family, which she was bringing up herself.

She was quite ready to acknowledge the inconsistency between her application for nurse training and her benefits status, and told me that she would withdraw her claim for benefits. However, I could only speculate that, some years earlier, the social and financial demands on her must have influenced her behaviour and health beliefs sufficiently for her recovery from the injury to be so slow and incomplete that she appeared to qualify for this benefit.

JF

HEALTH BELIEFS AND THEIR IMPACT ON DISABLEMENT

Health beliefs exist in all societies, and they influence our behaviour whether we are ill or not. They are the result of interpreting what we perceive from our senses in the light of expectations drawn from our experience and what we are told by others. Sometimes people will say that they did not know that they were ill until the doctor told them that they were. High blood pressure is a good example of this. Medical theory tells us that blood pressure which is elevated substantially above the norm puts the individual at greater risk of suffering a serious cardiovascular incident, such as a stroke or a myocardial infarction. However, there are believed to be no particular symptoms associated with higher than average blood pressure. In fact people with above average blood pressure are usually feeling very well – at least until they get this news! At this point, many people then start to feel that things are wrong with their body which conform to their *understanding* of what the high blood pressure might be doing to them. They may suffer headaches, exhaustion and throbbing in the head, all of which they will happily ascribe to their 'blood pressure.'

Effect of treatment delays on health beliefs

Sometimes employees will stay off work while waiting to have a procedure undertaken, such as an MRI scan or nerve conduction testing, or while waiting to see an NHS consultant. If there is a long time to wait, it is unlikely to be an emergency and is much more likely to have been ordered to provide reassurance. However, the delay can have the opposite effect. The employee may feel that they are terribly ill and fear a devastating diagnosis, or they may even feel that they are being neglected as a result of the delay. Yet the purpose of the investigation may simply be to reassure them that they do not have, for example, a serious back condition. Ironically, the enforced idleness of waiting may give them time to worry, and the worry itself may become the cause of incapacity – the employee may well 'worry himself sick', feeling that he is really sick and that his needs are being ignored. So it is always worth asking yourself (and if necessary checking with your patient's occupational health provider) whether a return to work pending completion of the investigation might be possible, perhaps with adaptation of their job, or temporary redeployment.

Effect of health beliefs on recovery

Pre-existing health beliefs will determine what a person feels about their illness, and it is often necessary to take these beliefs into account when treatment is being provided. Health beliefs will also strongly influence a person's recovery from a medical event which was responsible for an impairment. For example, an employee who suffers an acute attack of severe back pain may have an expectation that he should rest and refrain from work for a long period of time, as he has considerable life experience of colleagues being told exactly this over many years, before evidence-based medicine demonstrated that this strategy was unnecessary, and even harmful in some cases.

Health beliefs and language

The person's health beliefs need to be taken into account when drawing up plans for guiding them back to work. Chronic fatigue syndrome is frequently known to its sufferers by its earlier quasi-scientific name of 'myalgic encephalomyelitis.' This description went out of medical usage some years ago when science proved that the proposed mechanism was unsound. However, many sufferers and their carers continue to believe that the condition is due to a persistent virus infection (there is some evidence that virus infections can *trigger*, but not *cause*, the condition). Acknowledgement of (but not agreement with) such strong beliefs held by the individual may be instrumental in building a rapport with the employee, so that challenging them over the use of a particular name for a disease (which is at best poorly understood) may be unwise. Discretion is often the better part of valour, and building a positive rapport with the patient is essential when later on they may need convincing of the importance of participating in treatments such as cognitive–behavioural therapy, for pre-existing health beliefs also influence the person's response to therapy and rehabilitation.

So just as understanding the world of health beliefs and illness behaviours is as important to other aspects of primary care practice as evidence based-medicine, so it is also significant in relation to rehabilitation for work. Later in this book we will use the concept of flags to evaluate in more detail the place of health beliefs in recovery.

SICKNESS ABSENCE

Sickness absence is a specific form of illness behaviour, in which a person absents him- or herself from a work commitment or a number of other commitments, for a fixed period of time, on the grounds of illness which may be objective or which may be largely self-perceived. Usually a form of attestation will be offered (or sought by the employers), such as a sickness certificate signed by a GP after a particular number of days. In many cases, the outcome of the consultation which results in the issuing of a sick note will be determined by the patient, as most GPs regard their role as an advocate, and they feel that they have to support their patient. In any case, the types of illness which may be presented to the GP, namely short-term conditions such as diarrhoea, lethargy and stress, are difficult to challenge.

Expressing your concerns about sickness absence

As a GP you may well indicate your concerns about a certificate and retain control in what is otherwise a patient-led and directed consultation in a number of ways, perhaps by giving a short duration or a fixed date (i.e. a 'closed' certificate), or by using an ambiguous or even amusing diagnosis. For example, a GP recently admitted to a national newspaper that he had used the acronym TALOIA '15 times recently on certificates', and that TALOIA stands for 'there's a lot of it about'!

Use of a meaningless acronym such as this (or older ones such as 'plumbum pendulus') does send a witty and discrete message to the employee, the employer and the employer's occupational health provider (if there is one) that this absence is not about a life or death matter. Unfortunately, it risks further trivialising employers' views about GP certificates – which may bounce back on the GP when he is unable to get an employer to take him seriously on another occasion. However, the use of comments such as 'he *claims*', 'she *says*' or 'he *believes*' in factual reports commissioned by the occupational health provider conveys the sense that the comments are derived from his patient's remarks and, in a non-prejudicial way, implies that there is as yet no objective evidence to support such assertions.

Avoiding prejudicial terms

As a GP, you should be especially carefully to avoid using terms on sick notes which may later prove prejudicial. For example, the use of the term 'workplace stress' on a sick note should be reserved for those situations where you have sufficiently strong evidence to back up the claim. Simply repeating the term because the patient has used it, without further checking, risks the sick note being used as 'evidence' by solicitors and others – and you risk being asked at a later date to provide 'more evidence' to support the patient's opinion in court cases and claims, etc.!

Contributory factors with regard to sickness absence

There are many reasons why people 'go off sick', and it is rarely simply due to a bout of sickness. They may feel tired or unappreciated, or they may have travel difficulties which are highlighted by the illness. For example, a person with diarrhoea or dysuria is unlikely to come into work if they have to drive for 50 miles to get there, or if they work peripatetically, whereas another person who works from home or in an office which is adjacent to a toilet might well continue in work. However, if the employee feels stressed or undervalued, these feelings may well precipitate an absence that would not otherwise occur, whereas if they had been positively motivated they would take simple over-the-counter remedies and 'see how it goes.'

If an employee feels pressured by a bullying or over-enthusiastic manager, taking sick leave for a minor illness is an obvious way for that employee to consciously or sub-consciously re-establish control in a relationship where they feel that the power balance is becoming more unequal in the manager's favour.

WHAT FOLLOWS . . .

In Chapter 2 this book will continue with a discussion about why (in most cases) work is a health-promoting activity, and what happens when people 'go off sick.' Chapter 3 will then consider the principles and practice underlying return to work and rehabilitation. This is followed by an exploration of the role of primary care in return to work, first guided by a GP with special experience in this field in Chapter 4, and then by exploring the pathway that leads to incapacity and economic inactivity in Chapter 5, which is written by a senior lay occupational health adviser, who reflects on patient experience. In Chapter 6 the opposite paradigm is considered, namely how a person can be judged fit for (and to return to) work and, if so, what work. Chapter 7 considers the roles of the various professionals who can assist a practitioner in enabling return to work, and Chapter 8 contains a number of relevant case studies. Chapters 9 and 10 outline the formal limits within which we all work in this branch of medicine. In Chapter 9 the impact of social security rules and regulations is outlined, and Chapter 10 sets out the essential principles of law which operate in this area of medical practice.

FURTHER READING

Halligan P, Aylward M. *The Power of Belief.* Oxford: Oxford University Press; 2006.

Halligan P, Bass C, Oakley D. *Malingering and Illness Deception.* Oxford: Oxford University Press; 2003.

Waddell G. *Models of Disability.* London: RSM Press Ltd; 2002.

CHAPTER 2

Why does rehabilitation for work matter?

WORK AND HEALTH: THE HISTORICAL PERSPECTIVE

The need for labour

Hunter-gatherer societies depended on hunting wild animals and collecting nuts, fruit and berries for food. It was only with the development of agriculture that the requirement for labour emerged. Agriculture then tied mankind to the land and imposed a discipline on the active members of society to ensure that cultivation was sufficient to support greater populations than had been possible for hunter-gatherer societies.

Paid work and industrialisation

The greater population supported by cultivated land enabled society to sustain activity beyond that required for food production alone. Thus paid employment (e.g. 'the labourers in the vineyard') was already familiar in biblical times. As the opportunities for employment increased, so did the range of hazards to which workers were exposed. Industrialisation represented a further sophistication of the relationship between work and incentive, such that many generations of workers now moved to towns and across oceans in search of higher rewards, where they also found themselves at risk from new hazards such as smoke, heat, chemicals and powered machinery.

Fitness for work

The concept of keeping workers fit for employment existed in medieval monastic houses, where apothecaries grew and compounded drugs to keep monks and lay brothers fit for work and prayer. Later on, secular apothecaries were commissioned to treat the sick poor by public authorities under the Elizabethan Poor Law, so as to keep them fit for work and reduce the liabilities of the parish. Ultimately, in the early nineteenth century, these lay apothecaries blossomed into general practitioners when the apothecary profession merged with the man-midwives and absorbed a large number of ships' surgeons who had been made redundant by the end of the Napoleonic Wars and the abolition of slavery in 1807 (slave ships were required to carry a surgeon to keep the slaves fit for work, just as the naval surgeons treated the sailors of Nelson's 'wooden walls').

The need for certification

In the mean time, workers began to insure themselves through friendly societies against the financial risk of becoming unfit for work, thereby remaining independent of the parish and its coercive institutions such as the workhouse. However, like the parish, these societies developed their relationships with general practitioners, based on the treatment and rehabilitation of injured and sick members and gate-keeping access to direct payments. Certification of those unable to work became an associated (if unpopular) duty of GPs. In 1911, the health and welfare reforms of Lloyd George created the 'panel note' as we know it.

THE PHYSICAL AND MENTAL HEALTH NEEDS OF INDIVIDUALS OF WORKING AGE

It is self-evident that a certain amount of physical and mental health and fitness is necessary for a person to work, although experiences in wartime suggest that the human frame is capable of superhuman effort when required. Nevertheless, working when unfit (known as 'presenteeism') represents a risk both to the individual and to production, most obviously in the form of injuries, and the primary purpose of certification is to guard against presenteeism.

The ancients and work

The ancients generally regarded work as favourable and health-giving. Virgil believed that 'Work conquers all', and Galen described work as 'nature's best physician' and 'essential to human happiness.' Nevertheless, Hippocrates also gave us our first advice on presenteeism, namely that 'Hard work is undesirable for the underfed.'

Training and travel to work

The economic roots of our present complex society lie in the nineteenth century, where the relationships between consumers and industrialisation became established and led to other phenomena, such as travel to work and the concept of labour supply. It was no longer possible for work to be undertaken without qualifications or training, and individuals became identifiable by their trade or occupation, if they had one. However, this meant that a more complex relationship developed between labour and management, with the right people not necessarily in the right place. In 1911, the Lloyd George government introduced labour exchanges (a German concept) to bring together managers and labour supply. As the responsible minister, Winston Churchill ordered that the new exchanges be painted green, which is the 'colour of hope.'

Work role and society

Thus work is important to society, and it is work that establishes our place in society. Without employment it is impossible for outsiders to classify us socially, and it is largely our employment that, in adult life, moulds our experiences, hones our skills and creates at least some of our social circle. However, it is not possible for everyone to do what they enjoy. As Bertrand Russell remarked, 'Work is one of two kinds. One, moving particles of matter around at or near the earth's surface. Two, telling other people to do so. The first is unpleasant and badly paid. The second is enjoyable and well paid.' However, not everybody agreed, and Oscar Wilde wryly remarked that 'Work is the curse of the drinking classes.'

Epidemiology of worklessness

There is some evidence that work is becoming less satisfying to some groups of workers, especially older workers and those in the clerical and sales groups, which comprise a large part of the modern workforce. However, Waddell and Burton[1] noted that in public health terms, the risk of long-term worklessness is equivalent to smoking 10 packets of cigarettes per day, and is a greater risk than the most dangerous jobs on building sites or in the North Sea industries.

Public health

Recent years have seen increasing government interest in the epidemiology of worklessness and the public health risks of unemployment and incapacity. The Public Health White Paper of 2004 devoted a whole chapter to work and health, which pointed out that unemployment results in increased alcohol consumption and more smoking. It is also associated with weight gain and reduced physical exercise, despite the greater availability of time.

THE IMMEDIATE HEALTH EFFECTS OF REDUNDANCY

While working as an occupational physician in a shipbuilding town, I visited a chain store one evening to check the prices for a large television which my children wanted. I reckoned that I might get a bargain compared with the stores at home, but was surprised to see huge stocks at normal prices. The manager told me that when there was a redundancy programme at 'the yard', they always stocked up on large televisions. As the men facing redundancy attended their exit medicals, I enquired about their plans. Apart from the occasional dream of opening a bar in the Canary Islands or a chip shop in Whitby, most of them described plans for inactivity. You can understand a man who had worked for 30 years saying 'Put my feet up for six weeks', but this very action would put the 50-year-old at the back of the queue of 700 redundant men for the few 'good' jobs available in a town of 60 000 people. As the programme started, the young, fitter men took voluntary packages and migrated to construction jobs in southern England, leaving behind the older, less fit men, sometimes with disabilities (such as musculoskeletal conditions and hand–arm vibration disease). Before being named for compulsory redundancy (on better than voluntary terms), these tradesmen had been redeployed into unskilled jobs, and unsurprisingly a number of them 'went sick' before being made compulsorily redundant. At this stage, incapacity became a self-fulfilling prophecy, in that they needed to remain sick in order to retain their incapacity benefits, so is it surprising that they indulged in unhealthy behaviours?

JF

Overall, unemployment is associated with poorer psychological well-being, and with an increased incidence of self-harm, depression and anxiety.

LONGER-TERM ADVERSE HEALTH EFFECTS OF REDUNDANCY

When undertaking field work on health and work for a government department, I spent some time in a former coal and steel town in the Eastern Valleys. While counting the boarded up shops of what had once been department stores on quite a prosperous high street, I was stopped by a man who turned out to be a local councillor. 'They call it the northernmost outpost of the Ho Chi Minh trail', he said, 'More Vietnamese takeaways than anywhere else in the UK.' He told me that even the pubs had closed down, and that a lot of the men were constantly drunk on cheap cider which they bought from convenience stores. Their wives had taken the factory jobs which had been provided with regional aid. The men were reluctant to take these jobs, but would not keep house or cook either. As a result, many marriages broke up and the men lived alone or with elderly parents and existed on takeaways. A local researcher reported that an ex-miner had told him that he could not cope with factory work because it made him feel 'claustrophobic.' He had managed 20 years deep underground, but could not cope with the constant attention of the supervisor!

JF

There is growing concern that incapacity might be contributing to *worklessness* – where whole communities, often straddling generations, remain economically inactive. Ironically, in such communities it is the employed who may feel socially excluded from community activity, which may only occur during the working day.

SOCIAL EXCLUSION OF WORKERS

A post-office worker with a severe lower limb fracture was seen at a social security medical centre for assessment for incapacity benefit. He lived and worked in one of the 1960s 'new towns' which was populated by dwellers from slums cleared in a neighbouring city. However, many of the light industries which had been attracted by the (initially) subsidised factory units had moved on, and those that remained prided themselves on not recruiting local people. As a result, a workless culture reigned in the town. 'I am the only one in my street that gets up and goes to work in the morning. By the time I come home all of the social events have happened. Nobody does anything in the evenings – they can't, anyway, as there aren't even any buses. Everything happens in the day, which makes it quite lonely for me when I get home.'

JF

The Government has repeatedly returned to the theme of worklessness in communities. In 2005, a strategy for the health and well-being of working-age people called *Health, Work and Well-being – Caring for our Future*, was published. This has now been followed up (March 2008), with an in-depth study of the health of Britain's working age population, led by Dame Carol Black and called *Working for a Healthier Tomorrow*.

Is work healthy?

A major literature review was recently undertaken for the Department for

Work and Pensions by Waddell and Burton,[2] to answer the question 'Is work good for your health and well-being?'

This review confirmed that *employment* is generally the most important means of obtaining adequate economic resources, which are essential for material well-being and full participation in today's society, and that employment and socio-economic status are the main drivers of social gradients in physical and mental health and mortality. However, this was with the proviso that various physical and psychosocial aspects of work can also be hazardous and pose a risk to health.

Conversely, *worklessness* appears to be associated with poor health. There is strong evidence that unemployment is generally harmful to health, causing higher mortality, poorer general health, longstanding illness, poorer mental health, psychological distress and minor psychological/psychiatric morbidity. In addition, it results in greater demands on health services, due to higher rates of medical consultation, medication consumption and hospital admission.

Re-employment seems to improve self-esteem and general and mental health, and reduces psychological distress and minor psychiatric morbidity, roughly in proportion to the adverse effects of job loss. Although the evidence is less strong, there is a broad consensus across disability and employment professionals and interest groups that when their health condition permits, sick and disabled people, especially those with 'common health problems', should be encouraged and supported to remain in or to enter (or re-enter) work as soon as possible. This is because work is believed by them to be therapeutic, helps to promote recovery and rehabilitation, and leads to better health outcomes. Returning to work minimises the harmful physical, mental and social effects of long-term sickness absence and the risk of long-term incapacity. It promotes full participation in society, independence and human rights, reduces poverty, and improves the quality of life and well-being.

People who re-enter work after moving off benefits generally experience improvements in their income, socio-economic status, mental and general health and well-being. Those who move off benefits, but who do not enter work, are more likely to report deterioration in health and well-being.

Health risks of work

Although this study showed that the balance of evidence is that work is generally good for health and well-being, for most people there are three major provisos. First, the findings refer to average or group effects, and therefore should apply to most people to a greater or lesser extent. However, a minority of people may experience contrary health benefits from not working.

Secondly, the health benefits of work depend on its *nature* and *quality*. Further research is required to identify the physical and psychosocial characteristics of jobs and workplaces that are 'good for health.' Finally, the social context must be taken into account, particularly social gradients in health and regional deprivation.

Thus the most recent scientific study has confirmed the wisdom of the ancients – that healthy work is health-giving for most people. However, it is clear from the statistics for sickness absence and receipt of incapacity benefits that this view is not widely held in society, or indeed at present in the medical circles that are responsible for certification. So what happens to the individual?

WHAT HAPPENS TO A PERSON WHEN THEY 'GO OFF SICK': THE BREAKDOWN IN INTERNAL RESILIENCE

'Going off sick' is a complex process for most individuals who are resistant to changing their habits and going off sick. For most of us there are some parts of our work that we enjoy and others that we don't, but we put up with the total sum and get on with it. We are able to do this because of our internal resilience, which resists the establishment of illness behaviour. However, when our resilience is lowered (perhaps by persistent adverse changes in the workplace), the presence of a minor illness may overwhelm internal resilience and allow the establishment of illness behaviour, including absence. The process of overcoming internal resilience involves complex thought processes in which the individual considers the acceptability of absence, in work, social and family settings, and its effects on their earning capacity and their other responsibilities for the care of children and dependent adults. They may also consider the nature of the absence. For example, do they *have* to stay in bed or do they just have to stay inside the house, or do they even have to do that?

The power of belief and resilience

Clearly, a primary care advocate is well placed to influence the patient's resilience, and for the many centuries before active therapeutics emerged, this was how medical practitioners achieved clinical success. By involving yourself in your patient's dilemma, through the considered use of a sick note, you may be able to help them to control the breakdown in their resilience and perhaps enable them to get a brief but much needed rest. You might be able to help the person directly (or indirectly by dialogue with occupational health services) to resolve underlying concerns and issues. And by titrating their response through sick certification you could assist a dignified and sustainable return to work. However, uncontrolled use of the sick note may prevent the return of resilience and disempower your patient in their workplace, perhaps permanently. The power of belief generated by a highly respected professional is not to be sniffed at – but perhaps the context of the professional has to be taken into account in judging his power, as the following vignette by Professor Haslam demonstrates.

THE MAGIC SPONGE

It was one of the most horrific football tackles I have ever witnessed. I was medical officer to the local team, and flinched as one of our forwards fell to the ground with a sickening crunch. His ankle was at a pathological angle. He simply couldn't stand, and certainly couldn't walk.

I ran on to the pitch, took one look at the dreadfully swollen and excruciatingly tender ankle joint, and knew exactly what to do. Let's face it – any A&E doctor would agree that an injury like this needed an X-ray.

So I shouted at one of the spectators to order an ambulance, and totally disrupted the game – until the team manager came running over with a bucket and a sponge.

'For heaven's sake', he yelled at the player, 'Stop being such a wimp.' And with that he applied his magic sponge to the swollen ankle, and said those biblical words 'Now get up and walk', followed by a less than biblical descriptive noun.

And lo, he did. Groaning, limping, and then (incredibly) running. It was quite extraordinary. I felt completely and overwhelmingly outsmarted by the manager's magic sponge, but I still know that any doctor seeing an injury like this would have X-rayed and medicalised it.

So is there a lesson here for us general practitioners? Is the magic sponge yet another in the long line of alternative therapies? And whilst we are puzzling, just remember. He stood up, limped, ran, and scored. Endorphins are wonderful things.

Professor David Haslam
President of the Royal College of General Practitioners

WORK INSTABILITY

Everybody suffers occasionally from the catastrophic effects of an illness which stop them working, albeit briefly. Severe diarrhoea or fever due to an attack of influenza may physically prevent actual attendance at work briefly for even the most highly motivated of individuals. However, highly paid professionals may be able to continue sending emails from home or performing many of their tasks over the telephone. Return to work in such cases is generally rapid.

In other cases, the course of an absence is less straightforward and, in retrospect, perhaps more predictable. GPs may be perplexed by the repeated attendance of a patient with trivial complaints. There can be many explanations for this, but occasionally what follows is an eventual request for a sick note (or something else indirect, such as help with a relative or a prescription for impotence!). As a GP, you may be aware that the patient (to use an old-fashioned expression) is 'sickening for something', but the request for the sick note may be the first clue to the underlying agenda. For example, the patient may be attending repeatedly about a headache that doesn't go away or a cold that 'keeps coming back', but it is only on the third visit that the request for a sick note surfaces.

What you may have been observing is *work instability*. Work instability is more commonly described in the context of severe impairments caused by conditions such as multiple sclerosis and rheumatoid arthritis, where the individual struggles to meet their own or others' expectations at work. They may take repeated absences due to trivial causes which may not even be recorded as sickness absence – or they may take annual leave at short notice (known in some companies as 'floaters'). Work instability will be considered in more detail in Chapter 5.

The same presentation of frequent symptoms (that are difficult to explain) in relation to work can present in individuals without a severe impairment. Indeed they may or may not have a 'common health condition.'

Changing health or changes in the workplace?

In such cases the underlying impairment may be the person's work or it may be in their workplace. Working practices may have changed (e.g. the introduction of targets or piecework), or there may have been a major change in work conditions, such as the introduction of longer or fluctuating shifts or changes to arrangements for annual leave or pensions. What is common to such changes is that the employee – your patient – feels unable to influence the change, although it may well suit his colleagues as well as shareholders, managers and trade unions.

Talent-spotting work instability

This may enable you, as a primary care advocate, to support or empower your patient to respond to the underlying challenge. In later chapters, strategies to help you to do this with the aid of other professionals will be discussed.

But by 'going off sick' your patient will actually undermine their negotiating position. However, the identification of a relevant medical condition, such as hypertension, diabetes or peptic ulceration, may provide justification for referral to the company's occupational health provider. Even if the individual is not deemed to be covered by the Disability Discrimination Acts, a proactive approach may enable employment to continue with the establishment of a modification or adjustment to shifts, targets, hours or place of employment, just the same as if the impairment was due to one of the serious medical conditions identified above.

WHAT HAPPENS TO A PERSON'S LIFE IMMEDIATELY AFTER 'GOING OFF SICK'?

The domestic life of the individual changes as soon as they stop going to work. You may already have some experience of this with a long holiday!

❯ First, the habit of *getting up in the morning* is broken, and the person may also stop getting dressed properly, especially if they have acquired (perhaps in childhood) the health belief that convalescence from illness requires bed rest – or even the wearing of nightclothes for much of the day. If they are not getting up, the person doesn't need to wash their work clothes (or even themselves!), iron their shirts or polish their shoes.

❯ They may (depending on their illness) be less tired by nightfall, so may have *difficulty getting off to sleep*. They can then get into a cycle of sleeplessness, exacerbated by napping during the day, perhaps precipitated by watching daytime television!

❯ Their season ticket may expire and their car may need repairing or their licence renewing – *expenses which can be deferred* indefinitely into the future.

❯ While recovering, your patient may have acquired *extra domestic responsibility* for children or grandchildren, cooking meals or checking up on an elderly relative.

❯ Finally, while off sick, your patient's *outgoings decrease* as they no longer have to find money for lunch at the canteen, or for transport to work, or to pay for their suits to be dry-cleaned. Indeed they may actually receive a tax rebate!

So a number of changes in domestic life occur fairly quickly when a person stays off sick. In the workplace, the individual immediately avoids responsibility for whatever they were doing on the day they went off sick, and may have to be relieved more permanently of some of their more challenging work. These responsibilities will have to be transferred to a colleague, thus creating a feeling of guilt and fear of attitudes of hostility and exclusion from colleagues when the individual returns to work.

IMMEDIATE DISADVANTAGES OF BEING OFF SICK

There are also important disadvantages to being off work due to sickness.

›   While they are off sick, the employee loses the support of the daily *banter and craic* which is a normal part of our working lives. Colleagues become more distant, and invitations to social events such as retirement parties and Christmas outings may be overlooked.
›   The individual may *miss opportunities* for advancement or sideways moves to more desirable roles, including the chance to pursue vacancies that might withdraw them from a stressful job.
›   If the employee is feeling stressed by work or has a disciplinary process pending, they are *not in a position to defend themselves* or to safeguard their interests in the political environment which exists even in the most casual of workplaces.
›   More prosaically, the individual may also *miss out on material benefits* such as shift pay and piecework.

Overall, the absent employee has *voluntarily surrendered the social advantages accorded to them by employment*. Reminding them of these losses is a useful strategy which can be adopted when encouraging them to consider a return to work. The regaining of these lost social privileges can become a strong motivator for the individual, which a primary care advocate can use to advantage. In helping your patient to avoid becoming trapped in their illness and so unable to return to work, it will be helpful at this stage to consider what happens to them from the point of view of officialdom as they make the same journey through the 'welfare system.'

THE PATIENT JOURNEY IN SICKNESS ABSENCE

When a patient presents in your surgery requesting your support for taking sickness absence (or you suggest this), they will often mention the need for a form of attestation from you, by means of a certificate. It is not necessary (under state regulations) for you to provide an official medical statement until they have been absent for a week, and there a number of other certificates which are used at various stages of incapacity, as well as the familiar Med 3 (*see* Chapter 9). For an absence of less than a week, a certificate is not required, although occasionally employers demand one as they are required in law to pay Statutory Sick Pay (SSP), and may have doubts about the incapacity. If you choose to provide a sick note in these circumstances, you may charge your patient (or his employer) for it. However, in so doing you may be creating a rod for your own back, for far from creating a deterrent to the employer, your charges may actually gift to them a convenient way of deterring absence in their workers, by insisting on having a certificate for short absences!

If absence continues, your patient will continue to receive SSP for up to 28 weeks, and it is during this stage that you may receive a formal request from their employer (or the employer's occupational health provider) for a factual report to enable the provider to undertake an independent assessment. Such a request needs to be accompanied by a consent form signed by your patient. It is important to recognise that consent to provide a confidential report to a manager may later not be regarded by a court as consent that is freely given, but one which has been given under duress, so it is wise only to address your comments to the employer's occupational health practitioner and, if necessary, to insist on appropriate consent for this.

INFORMED CONSENT

I was asked to visit an employee at home who had been off sick for a long time. Unfortunately, I could not find the house, so I phoned the human resources department to ask if they would permit me to obtain a factual report from the person's GP, before trying again. 'We have one on file', I was advised, and in due course it arrived. Fully consented, it revealed intimate details of this man's terminal cancer and his treatment, but had been sitting in a file in a personnel office, for all the staff to read. The GP had not realised that in accepting consent from a human resources officer, his report might reach a wider audience and that a court might later judge it to be not freely given. And the GP himself could later find himself challenged by the General Medical Council for breaking confidentiality, because consent was neither freely given nor fully informed.

JF

Role of the employer's occupational health provider – if there is one!

Your patient may be reviewed in person by his employer's occupational health provider, in which case this is an opportunity for you to work together with the occupational health practitioner to help the patient to plan their return to work. Therefore it is important that at this point your comments are addressed to the occupational health professional, as at this stage normally the Jobcentre Plus office (formerly the Benefits Agency, Department of Social Security, or Department of Health and Social Security) will not even know that the employee is off sick.

Once Statutory Sick Pay ends, at around 28 weeks, the employer will suggest that your patient should apply for Incapacity Benefit, and the Jobcentre Plus office will only then become aware of them. You will know that they have reached this stage because you will be asked to complete a Med 4 form by your patient, and if this does not contain sufficient information, the Jobcentre Plus office will ask you to complete an IB113 form.

The Jobcentre Plus office will then refer your patient to their Medical Services contractor, who will scrutinise the claim information and decide whether your patient needs to be assessed in person by means of the Personal Capability Assessment, or whether they can be regarded as exempt because they meet one of the exempting conditions (*see* Chapter 9). If your patient needs to be assessed in person, they will be summoned to a medical examination centre where the assessment will take place, and you will be independently sent a letter stating the result of the assessment.

Appeals against decisions and assessments

If your patient is unhappy with the outcome of their assessment, they can appeal to the Independent Tribunal Service. However, normally, the Jobcentre Plus office will review such cases first. In either event it is not necessary for you as their GP to give any additional evidence – if this is required, you will be asked for it directly by the office. However, if there has been a *significant* change in diagnosis, you may be able to speed up the review process by offering your patient an appropriate explanatory letter. Although patients (and welfare rights organisations) can be very persuasive in asking you to supply more evidence, you may be wasting your time or building false expectations if you provide more reports or letters which have not been requested and which don't add anything new.

In those cases where your patient does not have an employer because they are unemployed, or the employer has refused to pay Statutory Sick Pay because they are a recent or casual employee, the whole of the above process will be carried out by Jobcentre Plus, usually with the involvement of their Medical Services contractor.

WHAT FOLLOWS . . .

Thus, in summary, economic inactivity appears to be associated with adverse experiences with regard to population health, and most people of working age appear to enjoy better health if they are able to remain in or return to gainful employment, assuming that they have health-promoting employment. Once the individual 'goes off sick', their life changes dramatically and they become subject to a number of perverse incentives which start to build progressively and can create a mountain over which they have to climb if they are to be able to return to work. In the next chapter we shall consider the barriers to recovery and how they can be overcome.

REFERENCES

1 Waddell G, Burton AK. *Concepts of Rehabilitation for the Management of Common Health Problems.* London: The Stationery Office; 2004.
2 Waddell G, Burton AK. *Is Work Good For Your Health and Well-being?* London: The Stationery Office; 2006.

FURTHER READING

Holland-Elliott K. *What About the Workers?* London: RSM Press; 2004.
Department for Work and Pensions. *IB204: A Guide for Registered Medical Practitioners;* www.dwp.gov.uk/medical/medicalib204/ib204-june04/ib204.pdf (accessed 8 March 2008).

CHAPTER 3

Detecting and dealing with the barriers to return to work

MODERN REHABILITATIVE PRACTICE

In this chapter we shall mainly concentrate on finding and responding to the barriers to return to work, but before doing that, we shall look at what constitutes the general principles of modern rehabilitation for work, namely:

- healthcare intervention
- increasing activity levels and restoring functions
- personal and psychological elements
- enablement and empowerment
- modified work.

Healthcare intervention

First, there needs to be timely and effective healthcare. As a GP, you should be able to either provide this or influence its timely supply through secondary care.

Increasing activity levels and restoring functions

Although specific exercise produces changes in physiological measurements, there is a more limited improvement in activity levels and return to work. Rehabilitation therefore needs to dovetail exercise into improved activity levels, leading to increased participation and social functioning. This is also true with regard to mental health problems, where increased physical activity improves depression and mental health. Programmes should increase the length of activity rather than allow it to be limited by symptoms. Increased activity improves the sense of well-being, confidence and self-efficacy, which in turn promotes compliance. Increased activity levels generally progressively reduce pain, subject to some ups and downs. Beliefs about rest and activity should include recognition of the therapeutic value of work.

Personal and psychological elements

Changing dysfunctional perceptions, attitudes and behaviour is central to the rehabilitation of many common health problems. Most approaches now combine cognitive–behavioural principles. Cognitive approaches focus on mental events, changing how people think about and cope with their symptoms, analysing their beliefs and what they do about them, and building confidence in their own abilities and skills. Behavioural approaches concentrate on changing illness behaviour, trying to extinguish observed illness behaviour by withdrawal of negative reinforcement such as medication, sympathetic attention, rest and release from duties, and to encourage healthy behaviour by positive reinforcement. The underlying principle is operant conditioning using strong feedback on progress. Training involves the patient's partner and family so that they continue the same management, and all health professionals involved in the patient's continuing care must take a consistent approach to change beliefs and behaviour and improve functioning.

Enablement and empowerment

Modern rehabilitation is all about rebuilding capacity. Enablement is an individual concept, and is about helping individuals to achieve goals which they have set for themselves. Empowerment is about encouraging people who may have become passive to demand what they require in order to recover and participate actively in citizenship. Along with demanding rights, disabled and sick people have to live up to their responsibilities. Enablement and empowerment are central to modern rehabilitation. Goals include:
> breaking the cycle of expectations and achievements
> building motivation, confidence and self-esteem
> changing self-image
> taking control of how they lead their own lives
> personal development
> accepting responsibility for contributing to the well-being of themselves, their family and their community.

Modified work

Individuals with common health problems may find their work difficult, painful or stressful. They may find it difficult to return to their normal duties. Adjustments to work tasks or the work environment, to reduce physical and mental stress, should facilitate early return, which is the basis for the provision of modified work. Whether this consists of adjustments to normal duties, gradual return to work or return to a different job, work adjustments need to be distinguished from notions that work is the cause of the problem and that a return to work will cause harm. Workplace adjustments must be firmly rooted in facilitation, and need to be temporary, a return to normal being the ultimate goal. Adjustments can be difficult to implement due to resistance from colleagues (sometimes as a result of jealousy) or managers (due to difficulty fitting in with existing processes and practices). For most people with common health problems it therefore needs to be emphasised that a return to normal work is perfectly feasible. It is unlikely that as a GP you will be able to safely and accurately suggest achievable adjustments inside the workplace. However, you should be able to trigger an occupational health review by a well-placed comment on a sick note. If the employer does not have a provider, your remark will encourage them to appoint one.

Further information on the concepts underpinning modern rehabilitation for work in common health conditions can be found in *Concepts of Rehabilitation for the Management of Common Health Problems* by Waddell and Burton.[1]

WHAT DO WE UNDERSTAND BY BARRIERS TO RETURN TO WORK?

As soon as your patient goes off sick, the barriers to a successful return to work start to build, and some of these result in implied secondary gain. The individual, although not unaware of these factors, is not necessarily motivated by them. However, the cumulative effect of a number of secondary gain factors can create a mountain which is difficult to climb even when the person has fully recovered. By talent spotting the barrier flags, you can help your patient to deal with the barriers and ensure a timely return to work. In this chapter, we shall first consider the flags themselves and how to identify them as barriers to a return to work, and we shall then suggest ways of using this knowledge to encourage a return to work.

SPOTTING THE BARRIER FLAGS

The flags are a concept which originally emerged in the 1990s in New Zealand as a means of screening for the risk of an individual with acute low back pain developing prolonged pain and disability, which would affect their quality of life and possibly result in job loss. The first important distinction was to separate the red flags, which require medical investigation and intervention, from the psychosocial yellow flags, where a broader range of interventions, not necessarily of a medical nature, are indicated to prevent chronicity.

THE FLAGS AND REHABILITATION FOR WORK

The concept of the flags has evolved within occupational and disability assessment medicine practice, in order to identify the presence of factors which may act as barriers to recovery and return to work in areas other than back pain. The original red flags for absolute medical factors and yellow flags for psychosocial factors have been expanded to identify barriers to a smooth return to work. The general practitioner or practice nurse is particularly well placed to spot the 'yellow flag' or 'blue flag' harmful health beliefs barriers as their patient transits an illness or injury, and the practitioner can then be poised to act to ensure a sustained return to economic activity.

THE FLAGS IN RELATION TO RETURN TO WORK

The flags provide a key framework in primary care to enable you to assess your patient and plan their return to work.

- *Red flags* are the conventional biomedical barriers, which usually require medical strategies.
- *Orange flags* represent co-morbidity (e.g. the patient with depression and back pain).
- *Yellow flags* represent health beliefs external to the workplace.
- *Blue flags* represent health beliefs within the workplace.
- *Black flags* represent financial barriers to return to work, including employment and insurance policies.
- *Chequered flags* represent social barriers to return to work.
- *Two or more flags can coexist* – for example, a person with 'red flag' back pain may also have 'yellow flags' or 'blue flags', i.e. harmful health beliefs.
- *Motivational interviewing* can be used to overcome the barriers to return to work once they have been identified.

Flags are non-prejudicial, and can also be readily be understood by involved lay people such as insurance case managers and human resource managers. Their role continues to evolve in rehabilitation for work practice, and the four colours of flags in common usage – black, blue, yellow and red – have been supplemented here by a 'chequered' flag, signifying social factors. A further flag (orange) for describing co-morbidity is also being studied at present, but its relevance to occupational health practice has yet to be determined.

RED FLAGS

Red flags are the absolute medical barriers to improvement after injury, impairment or illness. The investigation and actioning of red flags was the main reason why doctors and other health professionals became involved in the process of assessment and certification of unfitness for work in the first place. For example, in back pain, a red flag may be due to nerve root pressure symptoms or signs, such as weakness in the leg, alterations in sensation, or bladder symptoms, and can usually be confirmed by physical examination (e.g. alterations in tendon reflexes sensation) or investigations (e.g. MRI scans). By analogy, in mental health the presence of suicidal intent, thought disorder or cognitive impairment will dictate the need for urgent psychiatric assessment, or even inpatient treatment. Serious cardiac arrhythmias, joint/locomotor instability and investigation of possible cancers and fits are all examples of red flags, which generally result in a need for medical treatment, which may be surgical or conservative.

YELLOW FLAGS

Yellow flags represent psychosocial factors. In workplace health, yellow flags are usually regarded as those restraining health beliefs which *do not* relate to the workplace (the ones that do relate to the workplace are blue flags; see below). Beliefs about recovery and the effect of an illness or impairment affect people in different ways. Fundamentally, health beliefs are governed by psychological expectations, which in turn are influenced by experience and modified by education. GPs know their patients very well – over many years they get to know where they live, their families and their social interactions, and thus are well placed to anticipate their health beliefs. During recovery from illnesses, injuries and impairment, self-confidence is fragile, and is especially vulnerable to comments from those who are close to the patient, such as their partner, friends and relatives, or those whom the patient regards as important, such as medical and nursing practitioners and managers.

Language

The language used by health professionals (especially those in whom the patient has confidence, such as their primary care or specialist practitioner) is of considerable importance. Even today, doctors occasionally make dramatic and unhelpful *catastrophising* remarks without any evidence to support them – for example, 'You will *never* work again', 'Your X-ray is the *worst* that I have ever seen/*too bad* for surgery' or even '*severe* heart attack.' GPs will be aware of how such remarks are taken to heart by patients whose self-confidence has been undermined by long-term illness and dependence on others.

THE POWER OF CATASTROPHISING PROFESSIONAL LANGUAGE

During my early days in rheumatology I was confronted by a middle-aged former coalface worker who presented as a new patient with 'intolerable' back pain at my rheumatology clinic. He had not worked for more than 2 years, and was in receipt of invalidity benefit and attendance allowance. He came in supported (physically and otherwise) by his long-suffering wife, leaning heavily on a tripod. He displayed many of Gordon's [Professor Waddell's] signs, and all of his language revealed errant beliefs about back pain – he catastrophised, couldn't get a wink of sleep, painkillers were useless and he had lost faith in the medical profession.

During the taking of his history it transpired that at his first consultation with his GP following the initial episode of back pain after heavy lifting at work, the GP told him that he had received a report on the recent X-ray of his back. He [the GP] read the report silently to himself and said 'I'm not surprised, your back X-ray looks like the Battle of the Somme!' The patient told me that his father was in that battle and that 'it had been bloody awful.' On further questioning it was clear that he did not ask the GP for any further explanation. He knew then that he was 'doomed' and would end up 'crippled and in a wheelchair.' For the record, I got hold of his first X-ray and we discussed it together with another back X-ray for comparison – which was mine! I pointed out that his X-ray was not really different from mine. With some further primitive cognitive–behavioural therapy he did improve. He didn't return to work, but he became more mobile and physically active. We frequently referred to 'the Battle of the Somme', and he finally accepted that the GP's remarks were exaggerated and had caused him much worry and concern.

Professor Mansel Aylward CB
Director of the Unum Centre for Psychosocial and Disability Research, Cardiff

The influence of others

The perceptive primary care practitioner will also identify those unhelpful remarks made by the employee's line manager or colleagues. In the emergency services, for example, it is common experience for line managers to advise staff to 'stay off until you are *fully* recovered' or to state that 'we don't have any *light duties* here.' Such comments may appear well intentioned, but they also reflect internal politics. The reality may be quite different. For example, police officers who are staying off work due to stress commonly cite the pressure of paperwork, yet it may be that paperwork is exactly what an officer who is returning to duty after time off due to a neck or back condition or an abdominal operation is best able to do!

Getting the interpretation right

Yellow flags, being unhelpful health beliefs, can feed on themselves and considerably increase the delay in recovery. An employee who is anxious about their health and who has to wait for the result of a test will have their anxieties amplified and may well over-react to whatever they are told. This is especially true of X-ray findings, which may lead to catastrophising behaviour if not handled correctly. This phenomenon is often observed in cases where X-rays have been arranged as a result of an accident, perhaps under pressure from a solicitor, or abroad, where medical reports can appear alarming and even exaggerated.

BLUE FLAGS

Blue flags are the workplace barriers to recovery, and are often also due to psychosocial interactions, commonly between the individual and their direct line manager, or their work colleagues. When a person becomes ill and feels unable to continue attending work, their commitment may be undermined by any prevailing negative feelings associated with work. They may feel isolated by organisational re-structuring, or physical changes such as the introduction of open-plan offices. In recent times there have been rapid changes in ownership of companies, and staff may feel that the Transfer of Undertakings (Protection of Employment) (TUPE) regulations, far from protecting them, somehow reduce their value to that of a commodity.

Bullying

Another undermining effect in the workplace is that of bullying or harassment. In its worst form, this can actually be directed at encouraging the person to go off sick.

Often there is a breakdown in communication between the employee and their line manager, accompanied by a power imbalance, such that the employee feels threatened and intimidated. (However, this can go the other way, for it is equally possible for the manager to be the one who feels threatened, especially if their subordinates are older than they are or appear to be grouping together to undermine them.)

THE NEW HEADMASTER

'There is a hard way or an easy way – in my last school, the music teacher chose the hard way – he had a heart attack' [remark from a teacher, allegedly spoken by his new headmaster].

JF

Investigation of allegations

Conflict in the workplace, including bullying, may result in formal investigations. These may be instigated by the 'victim' (in which case they will be described as a grievance procedure), or they may be a disciplinary procedure instituted by a manager when there is an allegation of a breach of rules, regulations or procedures, or even following an accident. Sometimes both occur together and a grievance allegation follows shortly after the institution of disciplinary proceedings or, conversely, a disciplinary process is instigated following allegations of grievance.

BLACK FLAGS

Black flags are the *barriers to rehabilitation caused by financial circumstances.* These include employment conditions internal to work, such as periods of access to half pay or full pay, as well as external circumstances such as insurance policies which pay mortgages or loans during periods of incapacity, or which are triggered by disability and permanent ill health.

Entitlement to full pay or half pay

Directly employed public servants (including NHS staff, teachers, local government officers, civil servants and members of the emergency services) generally enjoy 'Whitley Council' conditions of service. This means that after a probationary period, they are entitled to full pay for the first 6 months of sickness, followed by 6 months on half pay. In certain circumstances, such as injury on duty, it can even be longer than this. During this time, a variable amount of attention will be paid to their absence by their managers. In some cases there will be a prompt referral to occupational health services, with conscientious implementation and follow-up of the recommendations. Regrettably, this is the exception, and in the majority of cases a long period of absence passes with little remedial action. This is unfortunate, because by the end of this time, even assuming that the initial cause of incapacity has been resolved, it is the absence itself which may have become the principal barrier to a successful return to work. For example, the school may need to make the teacher redundant so that a replacement can be appointed, a works department may have been reorganised to eliminate the post of the absentee, and so on. Analogous sick pay arrangements still apply in areas of the private sector which were once nationalised, such as ship building and the railways.

Insurance

Some employers share the financial risk of more generous support than Statutory Sick Pay by purchasing permanent health insurance for their employees. In return for fixed premiums, permanent health insurance providers accept the cost of meeting sick pay at a replacement level comparable with full pay. Unfortunately, this tends to have the same consequence as that described above, as public health insurance providers rarely provide active management of their smaller claims early on, when it is most feasible to achieve a return to work, which is why local health advocates such as GPs are best placed to intervene. Sometimes individuals themselves may have purchased such a plan, especially if they are self-employed.

Similar circumstances may exist with regard to patients who may have bought protection polices for mortgage or loan payments. GPs should be alert for requests to sign claim forms in addition to the usual sick note, as the patient may have a lot of debt on a credit card which is covered by such a policy.

Claims

In making a civil claim for damages, a litigant has to prove that the defendant owes them a duty of care in common law, and that he or she has suffered harm as a result of a breach of this duty of care. Such harm can include loss of earnings, so obviously a person who is making a claim against an employer, a public authority (e.g. due to tripping on a paving stone), a health professional or the NHS does not, in this respect, have a financial incentive to recover quickly. Furthermore, the 'no win, no fee system' is an incentive for lawyers to maximise the settlement, and staying off longer has this very effect. In addition, the plaintiff's lawyers may delay settlement until the last possible moment in case there is a precedent case which might influence the outcome in their favour.

One consequence of the move from company sick pay (with a replacement rate close to the employee's normal pay) to companies offering no more than basic Statutory Sick Pay is that it forces employees with high outgoings (e.g. mortgages and maintenance payments) to seek redress through the courts if they are unable to work because of an accident, so it is worth asking if your patient has seen a solicitor in the High Street or via their Trade Union.

Social security benefits

Social security benefits are a common 'black flag.' The most frequently encountered one is Incapacity Benefit, but a number of other benefits may also act as financial disincentives to recovery, including War Pensions, Prescribed Diseases, Disability Living Allowance, Industrial Injuries Disablement Benefits, and so on. In theory, Disability Living Allowance is an 'in-work', non-means-tested benefit, which is designed to support disabled people staying in work. In particular, the mobility component is intended to pay for transport such as a car or taxis.

However, claimants often perceive that a return to work will somehow reduce their chances of achieving or retaining this or other benefits. The need to fulfil a prospective test of 3 or 6 months may be a factor contributing to this perception. Housing benefits and other means-tested benefits, such as Income Support Disability Premium, can be very significant components of the income of the lower paid, especially if they have substantial family responsibilities, and may be a powerful black flag.

Secondary gain and volition

The above account implies that there are frequently factors other than recovery and illness involved in a patient's return to work. This is not to imply that, because of these factors, individuals do not wish to recover and return to their responsibilities, including their financial independence. However, the accumulation of financial disincentives creates a virtual mountain, which the individual needs to feel confident to climb before they can return to work. Obviously, the difficulty they may experience in returning to any of these benefits, insurances and allowances should a return to work be unsuccessful will influence them and thus their ability to recover.

DOES MALINGERING EXIST?

Earlier in my career I worked on the social security 'front line' in Liverpool, which was then infamous as the European capital of sick absence. Very few of the claimants were malingering – that is, were fraudulently exaggerating their symptoms and signs.

Occasionally a claimant drove away in the cab of his taxi, but most people were older, overweight, and lacking in the confidence necessary to return to work, with diagnoses like back pain or depression. In many cases their job had changed or disappeared, but they were usually capable of doing some work, if given the right support.

Very occasionally, however, frank malingering is encountered. I was sent by an insurance company to assess a manual worker, in his home, who had been absent for many months with back pain. Home was the flat above a pub where his wife was named as licensee. As I crept upstairs, past piled up crates of beer, his wife shouted 'When the doctor has finished with you, can you come and move these crates of beer into the bar for me? You know I can't lift them.' It turned out to be quite a brief visit, and the report was not long either – the patient and I agreed that he had now made a full recovery and he would be returning to work very shortly!

JF

SOCIAL FACTORS: THE CHEQUERED FLAGS

Occupational health professionals will be very familiar with a series of social factors which can act as barriers to return to work. Joy Walker, a senior nurse manager, suggested that these should be called chequered flags because they constitute a warning. They include:

❯ *Carers' responsibilities*:
  - for a disabled or sick partner, elderly parent, or child
  - providing first-line or back-up childcare for grandchildren or children, or taking them to or from school.
❯ *Retirement preparations*:
  - partner already retired
  - pre-retirement removal – employee nearing the end of their career chooses to move further away from work to a retirement location, but at the cost of a longer commute at the end of their career when they are least fit for this
  - overseas property purchase – the overseas property owner is dependent on cheap flights, and may visit their property for long spells of convalescence during sickness absence.
❯ *Civic and social responsibilities*:
  - school governors
  - councillors (especially during the mayoral office)
  - tribunal members.
❯ *Other commitments outside usual work*:
  - second jobs

- overtime
- trade union activities
- extramarital affairs or marriage breakdown.
- hobbies – e.g. amateur musicians

RECUPERATION OVERSEAS

A health professional in his early fifties was referred to an occupational health consultant after almost a year's absence. During this time, various interventions had taken place, but it remained unclear exactly what the diagnosis was and whether a permanent 'cure' had been obtained. The individual had lost their confidence and appeared older, but not sick, and when faced with the real prospect of capability dismissal (on expiry of sick pay), he immediately requested a return to work part-time.

On closer questioning, it appeared that he spent a large part of his absence in his Spanish property 'because the sun always makes you feel better.' His manager was reluctant to accept him back at work in case he went off sick again, because a return would trigger entitlement to further sick pay. The consultant therefore suggested a return to work part-time, i.e. just Mondays, Wednesdays and Fridays, 'so that he would have the opportunity to recover in between,' He had actually requested to work the three days together, presumably so that he could go abroad for breaks in between. The manager agreed to review the position after 6 months 'to see how he was coping.' Thus an incentive was created for the returnee to concentrate on his recovery, while leaving any 'hidden agendas' without discussion.

JF

ASSESSING DISABILITY

Consistency and compliance: is the cause of the absence 'genuine'?

When an employer asks you (and often tells you his own view!) whether the cause of the absence is 'genuine', he is usually referring to his subjective understanding of the robustness of its justification. In fathoming the answer to this question, the two most useful concepts to consider are consistency and compliance. In assessing disability, you are measuring *consistency* in the absentee's functioning to detect whether the restriction in their behaviour is consistent across their whole lifestyle. You may also be looking for evidence of *compliance* with treatment recommendations, which will confirm their commitment to their own recovery. Two particular components which are helpful in assessing disablement will now be explored, namely *taking a history of a typical day* and *functional observation*.

Taking a history of a typical day involves asking your patient to describe to you their typical day from the moment they get up in the morning until they retire. Get them to describe what time they wake and get up, dress and wash, how they prepare breakfast and for whom, and how they pass the morning, and so on, throughout the day. The purpose is to find out the exact level of functioning of your patient in different social arenas. Ensure that they tell you about any variability in their condition.

This approach is not intended to 'trip them up' or to detect malingering. Rather its aim is to map out your patient's confidence and functioning in different areas of their life. You may discover that their social confidence is returning faster in some areas of their life than in others. For example, they may be able to sit at their keyboard and play computer games, but are fearful of returning to work altogether or of getting upper limb pain if they return to computer work. If they have a dog, they may be able to go for long walks, perhaps even across uneven ground, so record how often and how far they walk.

Taking a history of a typical day should help to reveal to you the presence of adverse health beliefs which will need to be addressed, perhaps by yourself (e.g. 'I'm pleased to hear that you are now able to manage to play computer games *most* afternoons, so perhaps you are near to being ready to get back to work part-time'), or more formally by engaging cognitive–behavioural therapy.

USING THE TYPICAL DAY IN OCCUPATIONAL MEDICINE

Disability assessment methods can contribute to traditional occupational medicine as well as return to work, especially where there is the possibility of secondary gain. In assessment of hand–arm vibration syndrome, the individual may be aware that they might be eligible for compensation if they are unable to work in their trade, but most also want to continue in these trades, which are often well paid. Thus there is an incentive for exaggeration or minimising of their symptoms which may be difficult to elicit via a traditional occupational history. However, by exploring a 'typical day', it might be possible to detect functional limitations. For example, a heavy engineering worker claimed to be able to use his tools normally, despite sensory impairment that was demonstrable on examination. When asked how he spent his evenings, he declared 'drinking pints of Guinness – if they don't slip out of my hand.' He then admitted that his sensation was so poor that he could not grip a cold pint glass, and furthermore that he taped up the trigger on his hand-held drill because he could not grip it either – 'like all the other buggers on the night shift', as he ruefully remarked.

The drill weighed several kilograms and was being used on a scaffold at least 20 feet above the ground, and thus constituted a considerable risk to his colleagues who were working below him.

JF

Functional observation supplements a formal clinical assessment. We are all familiar with the situation where it is difficult to assess an individual objectively due to subjective or reactive responses on their part, such as guarding. For example, on formal assessment of straight leg raising it may appear as though almost no straight leg raising is possible in someone with simple back pain, but you may observe the same individual sitting upright on your couch with their knees flat without any apparent discomfort. This does not mean that they are malingering – it simply means that their function is different when they are distracted from being part of a formal assessment in association with their work. Thus a great deal can be gleaned from collecting your patient from the waiting room, noting aspects of how they get on and off the couch, checking politely whether they need help from the nurse attendant with undressing and dressing, and observing them as they leave you and walk out to their car.

Behavioural symptoms

Professor Gordon Waddell has studied low back pain extensively from a scientific, clinical and behavioural point of view. His studies identified seven forms of non-anatomical or behavioural symptoms which were distinct from the common mechanical symptoms of back pain:
- pain at the tip of the tailbone
- whole leg pain
- whole leg numbness
- whole leg giving way
- complete absence of any spells with very little pain in the last year
- intolerance of or reactions to many treatments
- emergency admission to hospital with simple backache.

(For further details, readers are referred to his book entitled *The Back Pain Revolution.*[2])

Although these non-anatomical symptoms have been evaluated in the specific context of back pain, they can with a little imagination (and anatomical understanding!) be considered by analogy in other contexts, such as upper limb disorders or even anxiety/depression.

Non-organic or behavioural signs

Professor Waddell has also developed a set of clinical *signs* which predominantly reflect on the patient's behaviour, although they are also vulnerable to observer bias.

> Tenderness which does not conform to expected musculoskeletal anatomy. In the case of low back pain this can be superficial or deep (non-anatomical).

> Simulation tests in which an apparent test is performed which appears to stress part of the body, but in fact does not do so. For example, pressing down on the skull will cause physiological neck pain, but not pain in the lower back, and if the patient volunteers painful sensations in their back, this is a behavioural sign. Similarly, a patient who is standing can be asked to rotate their lumbar spine. In so doing, they will actually move their hips, so if they volunteer pain in their back, this must be a behavioural sign.

> Distraction tests can be as simple as noting how easily the patient gets on and off the couch or dresses and undresses, compared with formal examination, or can involve comparing straight leg raising when they are lying on a couch or sitting up or forward on the edge of the couch while distracted by testing the reflexes, discounting the fact that there is an anatomical advantage of 20 degrees when sitting.

> Regional weaknesses or sensory changes, which do not conform to known anatomical patterns.

Once again, these tests which are designed for evaluating low back pain can, with imagination, be adapted for other parts of the anatomy.

GETTING AROUND THE BARRIERS: USING THE FLAGS TO HELP PATIENTS TO PLAN THEIR REHABILITATION/RETURN TO WORK

Awareness of the flags equips you as primary care advocate to help your patient to avoid getting locked into a state of permanent incapacity and economic inactivity which would adversely affect their health for the rest of their life through impoverishment. There are no general rules, but here are a few specific tips.

When issuing certificates and reports

Always be cautious about certification, and pay particular attention to the following.

❭ Timing issues.
- *Issue certificates which are time limited.* Giving a definite time limit imparts a subtle message to the patient.
- *Don't issue overlong certificates.* If you write '13 weeks', your patient will believe that they won't or can't improve within the foreseeable future. Don't ever be persuaded to write 'until further notice' or 'UFN', unless the employee has incurable cancer or has entered the terminal phase of a severe condition such as motor neuron disease.
- *Issue certificates more frequently as the employee improves.* Coming back for a certificate after just a few days creates another opportunity to remind the employee that they are improving, even if they are not initially convinced about this!

❭ Wording issues.
- *Do not exaggerate (or tell lies)* by using diagnoses which you could not defend – if necessary in court.
- *Be direct.* Make it clear to your patient that you are only signing for what you have evidence for.
- *If you cannot agree with your patient's claims, avoid direct confrontation* by using euphemistic and 'vague' diagnoses such as 'nervous debility' and 'neurasthenia', which have stood the test of time and will convey a suitable message to an adjudicator or claims manager.

❭ When completing medical reports:
- *Use words like 'says'* or *'claims'* if that is all the evidence which you have to support a patient's claim.
- *Communicate your patient's compliance* with your instructions or not, to demonstrate whether they are cooperating with you and other health professionals in promoting their own recovery.
- *Reflect on the consistency (or lack of it) of the patient's behaviour* across a number of dimensions of their life, without being unduly challenging. For example, you might be able to comment on how they have successfully followed up your suggestions to take up a hobby or exercise again, or to take a holiday.
- *Complete an RM7 form* or make a remark on a sick note such as 'Occupational health opinion would be helpful.' Don't suggest light duties. This approach only works when the absentee has applied for Incapacity Benefit on expiry of their Statutory Sick Pay or Company Sick Pay.
- *Be open with you patient* – to avoid compromising your doctor-patient relationship you can say to them that you are not an expert in return to

work matters and you need a second opinion. Put like this, your patient is unlikely to argue with you.

HANDLING THE PATIENT WITH UNHELPFUL HEALTH BELIEFS IN PRIMARY CARE

- Be courteous and polite, even if you believe that the patient may be exaggerating.
- Avoid direct confrontation and prejudicial comments – a court or solicitor may ask for your records, and these may undermine your professionalism.
- Do be open and direct, though, making it clear that if asked for a report, you can only report on what you have evidence for.
- Use positive language, conveying an expectation of recovery, such as 'You seem much better' or 'Now you can do this and this . . .'
- If you feel that your patient is not working as positively towards their recovery as the medical evidence might suggest they are capable of doing, they may 'need encouragement.' If this is the case:
  - encourage your patient to participate socially, even going on holiday or playing golf, but as a definite part of returning to normal work activity
  - recommend exercise, which may be physical (e.g. walking, gym, swimming) if they have a psychological condition, or mental (e.g. quizzes, films, books, card games) if they have a physical condition which has undermined their confidence
  - recommend 'rehabilitation at home', such as DIY activities as a preparation for a return to work activity, so that the patient builds up their resilience
  - make use of 'accompanying persons', such as the patient's partner, who will reinforce your messages when they have left your consulting room.

Dealing with the red flags

With red flags, the emphasis needs to be on supporting your patient in their investigation, treatment and recovery process, while encouraging them not to burn their boats with regard to a future return to work.

- *During investigations.* It may be possible for your patient to return to work (perhaps through liaison with occupational health or human resources professionals) pending investigations or surgery. In such a case, the certificate can be annotated with this recommendation. This avoids the patient using up their sick pay provision – and their credit with colleagues!
- *Red flags are not necessarily permanent barriers to work.* Red flags may be absolute medical barriers to improvement at a particular time, but *they*

need not be permanent. For example, serious mental health conditions (even with suicidal intent) are likely to result in complete recovery, enabling the patient to return to their usual occupation, after formal occupational health assessment, although a recurrence in the future is a strong possibility.

❱ *If a serious diagnosis is sustained*, many people wish to continue working for as long as they can, for work is usually a social identifier of normality.

❱ *Facilitating rehabilitation of the patient.* You may be able to encourage your patient to see a rehabilitative professional. This will be a physiotherapist for a physical problem, or a talking therapist (i.e. a psychologist, counsellor or possibly an occupational therapist) for a non-physical problem. To do this, you may need to move mountains to engage one of the more reluctant parts of the NHS on their behalf. However, in some parts of the UK, access to rehabilitation professionals is possible for individuals who are off work due to sickness and claiming (or about to claim) incapacity benefits through the Condition Management Programme (CMP) of 'Pathways to Work' at the job centre. Normally, this is offered at a regularly scheduled work-focused interview (wfi); however, you can suggest that your patient seeks a wfi to discuss participation in the CMP.

❱ *Redeployment.* Even if complete recovery does not occur, red flags do not necessarily constitute an absolute barrier to further employment, as it may be possible to apply an adjustment to the working circumstances, which will enable your patient to continue in their employment. For example, a labourer with low back pain due to a herniated lumbar disc may be able to return to work as a depot clerk, where he can move around. Similarly, a trained nursery nurse working as a family support worker who develops ulcerative colitis might be able to cope with working in a day nursery, where she has access to a toilet, or she might be able to take 'office-type' nursing work (e.g. in a call centre). Such adjustments may be available under the Disability Discrimination Act (*see* Chapter 10), in which case the employer or manager will form a view as to whether they are 'reasonable' or not. However, with consultation, many employers are willing to offer adjustments to valued employees who do not meet the Disability Discrimination Act definition (*see* Chapter 8 for more examples). You will need to exercise some caution in pressing for redeployment, as a manager may say that none is possible. In such circumstances, your patient may find him- or herself made redundant if you have previously suggested that they are unfit for their previous post.

> *Achieving workplace adjustments.* From primary care, you cannot directly facilitate a workplace adjustment, as normally this will require a health professional such as an occupational therapist or case manager to conduct an assessment of their workplace. However, if their job is under threat and they apply to their local job centre requesting an assessment under 'Access to Work', they will normally be entitled to such an assessment. Their employer will then be expected to pay for the implementation of the adjustment up to a certain figure.
> *Never forget that the flags are not mutually exclusive,* and that a patient with red flags can also have blue, yellow and black ones!

Dealing with the yellow flags

In occupational medical practice, the yellow flags are particularly difficult to deal with, especially if a collusive relationship has developed between the patient and their GP or specialist. However, a primary care practitioner is well placed to influence the long-term outcome. He or she will have long experience of the patient, their expectations and experiences, and should have a shrewd idea of their health belief systems and motivators. They may have previously shared some of these, and the practitioner should have intimate knowledge of the patient's family and friends and may have visited their home. Above all, the patient is most likely to have trust in their practitioner, who will be crucial to the evolution of health beliefs.

Thus you may be able to anticipate the effects of illness or disability or even detect such an illness coming on – for example, if they attend several times with an illness that just doesn't get better (like a cold or cough) before asking for a sick note. This phenomenon (described earlier as work instability) will be discussed in more detail in Chapter 5.

However, in many cases you should be able to steer them towards brief psychological interventions based on positive thoughts, which may well be available from the Job Centre through 'Pathways to Work' locally, if not from the NHS.

Preventing harmful beliefs from becoming persistent

As you are their primary care advocate, your patients will rate your advice highly, and you will probably see them frequently, if only to give them a certificate, as they await their turn for specialist investigations. It is important to see this as an opportunity and not a burden. If your patient informs you that they will have to wait 3 months for a scan, it may be tempting to write a line for 13 weeks. However, in so doing you forgo the regular opportunity to influence their health beliefs in favour of a return to work.

By seeing your patient regularly and perhaps observing and drawing attention to their functional recovery, you may even render some investigations irrelevant by the time they are due to take place. Alongside your special knowledge of your patient and their family and environment, time is a really valuable tool for reviewing and considering your patient's recovery (as in other areas of primary care practice). People commonly believe that they cannot work when they are disabled or ill, and that they cannot return until they *fully* recover, whereas in fact neither of these beliefs is true.

Rebuilding confidence

Returning to the sometimes challenging environment of employment requires considerable self-confidence, and the individual will be uncertain as to their welcome by their managers and colleagues. It is therefore important to avoid making careless or undermining remarks, as this can be crucial for self-confidence. Simple acts, such as suggesting that your patient goes out, will prevent them losing confidence. Making sure that your patient keeps in contact with their workplace is important. Sometimes going on holiday can be a good way to rebuild confidence and at the same time get used to travelling and meeting deadlines again.

TAKING A HOLIDAY

An employee had been off sick for a long time, and his illness did not seem to be improving. He was clearly feeling a lot better, but did not yet have the confidence to return to his trade. I was seeing him monthly, and tentatively suggested that he should consider taking a holiday. At the following monthly appointment he said that his son had offered to take him abroad, and he asked me whether that would be okay.

I expressed immediate approval, but advised him to inform the human resources department. Somewhat taken aback at first, he smiled when I pointed out that this was a small town and it would better for him to tell the human resources managers than to risk allowing his gossipy neighbours to inform them. I suggested that he could say that the 'occ doc' had recommended it, and he jumped at this idea.

As he walked to the door, I also suggested that he should attend for an appointment on his return, when I would get him an easy driving job (on basic pay). Unsurprisingly, he recovered and was back in his trade (and back earning his bonuses) within 3 months!

JF

However, positive remarks made by primary care advocates are equally important in building confidence. These need not be challenging, for over a period of weeks, it is possible for a GP or practice nurse to work with the patient to rebuild their confidence, such that they are able to cope with the psychological demands of returning to their workplace, perhaps assisted by an adjustment negotiated with their manager, via the occupational health service.

Awaiting investigations

Waiting for an investigation such as an MRI scan can undermine the patient's belief that they are actually recovering (or are not seriously ill). The fact that they may have to wait months for such an investigation may paradoxically increase their anxiety as unhelpful health beliefs take over. They may believe that 'The doctor must think that I'm very seriously ill if he has ordered this expensive investigation' and that 'The NHS is failing to provide this test early enough, and I will get worse and need a wheelchair.'

Thus waiting may compound the absentee's anxiety, and they may seek alternative provision in the private sector, where the language used is sometimes less direct than that utilised in the NHS, and patients may be told more details than they can actually understand. In many cases the person can safely return to work (perhaps on modified duties) while such investigations (or even operations) are awaited, and this may be a good way to boost confidence and avoid the development of harmful beliefs. You may suggest this on the medical certificate by stating 'Can return to work on modified duties pending surgery or investigations.' If you are uncertain about which duties these would be, you can add 'as advised by occupational health service.'

Interpreting specialist language

These days, medical reports are often shared with the patient and may cause alarm which builds unhelpful health beliefs. Thus a report of 'cervical or lumbar spondylosis' may be misunderstood by the patient as confirming their worst fears of having a crumbling spine which will result in paralysis, rather than being simply an expression of their chronological age. Especially florid language may follow a consultation in some Mediterranean countries. As the patient's primary care practitioner, it is important that you help them to understand and interpret these findings in a realistic fashion. You are well placed to prevent such occasions from turning the patient into a victim and a chronic invalid by interpreting such findings with sense and sensitivity!

Dealing with the blue flags

The blue flags are the most difficult ones for primary care advocates, who will have little direct contact with or knowledge of the workplace, and even more limited influence. Therefore the first principle must be to do no harm.

Comment with caution and only with objective knowledge

Only issue statements that you can fully justify, and avoid getting drawn into conflicts from which it could be difficult to extricate yourself.

Be careful about citing 'stress'

Although the word 'stress' is not a medical term, it can provide an acceptable euphemism for anything from minor mental ill health conditions to frank psychosis. However, you should avoid prefixing 'stress' with 'workplace', unless you have evidence that would satisfy a court.

It is always a good idea to remember that because stress is not a medical term, a court might later ask you to define your patient's condition in true medical terms. If you cannot give a medical diagnosis, perhaps you should reconsider your use of this term. However, you can indirectly imply a sense that your concern focuses on your patient's workplace by using descriptions like 'anxiety/depression – no domestic stressors apparent.' Similarly, you could make a suggestion of workplace counselling or mediation to a human resources officer if you feel that there is a specific problem between an employee and their line manager.

Preparing your patient for a return to work

To prevent your patient's incapacity from becoming permanent, it is a good idea to continue to treat them as though they are returning to work, even if they clearly hope (or even intend) that they will not do so. Ensure that they keep in contact with their workplace. Suggest that when they are ready to return, they should ask someone to accompany them into work on the first day. This could be a friend or colleague or a trade union official, as 'the factory gates' can become a huge barrier.

Hostility in the workplace

The common result of hostility in the workplace is that negative expectations about the workplace are generated which undermine the person's belief in their ability to recover. It is also possible for a primary care practitioner to become unwittingly drawn into conflicts which result from such hostility in the workplace, particularly with regard to grievances, disciplinary procedures and requests for modified duties. This can be a problem, as you are unlikely to have any *objective* knowledge of the patient's workplace.

Going off sick prior to investigations

Sooner or later your patient will have to deal with workplace issues and get on with the rest of their working life. Therefore signing a sick note stating 'stress' may not be helpful in the long term, for it stalls the process, and leaves your patient excluded from the only place where the issue can be resolved, namely the workplace! While absent your patient cannot defend him- or herself, and other parties may also become stressed, especially as a prolonged delay makes it more difficult to recall events.

Fitness for a hearing

Eventually the formal process will have to be concluded, so the manager may seek an occupational health view on whether your patient is capable of participating either in person or via a written submission or a 'friend.' In such circumstances, fitness to attend a hearing will be judged at a lower level than fitness to attend work, and will focus on whether your patient has the ability to understand the allegations, whether they can distinguish right from wrong, whether they can understand and follow the proceedings (if necessary with extra time and written explanation), and so on. Therefore it might be prudent to consider these questions before issuing a certificate in the circumstances of a formal disciplinary or grievance process. However, if you consider that your patient's mental state is so vulnerable that suicide is a serious risk, you will be taking appropriate action, and short-term certification may be part of this.

Light duties

Quite often, a patient who has been absent from a physical occupation for some time may ask their GP if they can be certified 'fit for light duties.' Some employers are happy to accede to this advice (whatever it means!), especially when an employee has a heavy job and is convalescing from surgery. In other cases, such a sick note can cause a supervisor or middle manager to become incandescent with rage, as the suggestion that any of the duties in their management span may be 'light' will be regarded as highly provocative! Only an occupational health professional who is familiar with the culture of the company will be able to pick their way through these politics, so it is more prudent to state exactly what tasks the employee cannot do (e.g. no bending, or lifting of weights over 12 kg). If you don't feel confident about advising in this amount of detail, suggest on the note that your patient is reviewed by the company's occupational health practitioner with a view to making workplace adjustments.

Dealing with the black flags

Black flags, being financial, are particularly difficult to deal with. However, because these flags are often characterised by timing issues, this does create an opportunity for a primary care advocate to exert influence in various ways.

End of full pay/half pay

Public services workers will tend to have a period of full pay, which changes after some months to half pay, and then later to no pay. So as your patient approaches these periods of absence, they may be more receptive to efforts to help them back to work by, for example, counselling them to seek an interview with their human resources manager or recommending an occupational health referral on the medical certificate.

Insurance claims

These claims usually require verification by a treating practitioner, when you can discuss recovery plans. By contrast, simply signing the form in the absence of your patient may give an unconscious signal of your approval of their continued incapacity.

Risk of dismissal

It is a mistake to assume that just because a lengthy period of sick pay is tolerated, dismissal is unlikely. In fact, once sick pay has been exhausted, there may be no job left to return to, and your patient can be dismissed on capability grounds at this stage. It is always worthwhile reminding your patient of this eventuality.

Chequered flags (i.e. social factors)

As the patient's primary care advocate, you will be especially aware of these factors – more so than other professionals, especially those in the workplace. And you can use this knowledge to your patient's advantage by helping them to manage their convalescence. However, it is important that you remain in charge of their programme and ensure that it remains focused on a return their normal work, and does not drift. Some examples of approaches to this are listed below.

❯ Suggest that they go to their Spanish apartment to recuperate, but set a deliberately prescribed length of time, perhaps by a time-restricted certificate, so that they have to return to see you and are not tempted to languish when they get there.

> You may also discretely use your knowledge of their family commitments to encourage them to return to work as an exit strategy from exploitation (e.g. 'It was a good idea to look after the grandchildren to build your confidence, but I can't keep certificating you to do that').

> You may use your knowledge of their outside commitments, such as hobbies, civic duties or a second job (which they may be continuing with) to encourage them to find ways of returning to work.

THE FLAGS IN PERSPECTIVE

The flags provide a good structure for understanding the barriers to recovery and how to find ways to overcome them. They provide a common language which can be understood by the many health and other practitioners involved in the art and science of rehabilitation for work. They also provide a clear place for the particular contribution which medical and health practitioners can make (i.e. diagnosing and managing the risks of red flags). However, they also provide a structure whereby all of those professionals whom work-incapacitated employees meet on their journey can exert an influence. In Chapters 4 and 5 the journey of your patient/employee will be followed from the perspective of a GP and a lay occupational health adviser working in primary care.

REFERENCES

1 Waddell G, Burton AK. *Concepts of Rehabilitation for the Management of Common Health Problems.* London: The Stationery Office; 2004.

2 Waddell G. *The Back Pain Revolution.* Edinburgh: Churchill Livingstone; 1998.

FURTHER READING

Goodwill J, Chamberlain A, Evans C, editors. *Rehabilitation of the Physically Disabled Adult.* 2nd ed. Cheltenham: Stanley Thornes; 1997.

Halligan P, Aylward M. *The Power of Belief.* Oxford: Oxford University Press; 2006.

Halligan P, Bass C, Oakley D. *Malingering and Illness Deception.* Oxford: Oxford University Press; 2003.

Malleson A. *Whiplash and Other Useful Illnesses.* Montreal: McGill-Queen's University Press; 2003.

Waddell G, Aylward M. *The Scientific and Conceptual Basis of Incapacity Benefits.* London: The Stationery Office; 2005.

CHAPTER 4

Primary care and rehabilitation for work

This chapter considers sickness certification and incapacity for work specifically from a general practice perspective. Although GPs often get a bad press with regard to their supposed disinterest in sickness certification, and are sometimes blamed for continuing high rates of Incapacity Benefit (IB) claims, there is actually widespread interest in the topic at all levels from undergraduate medical students to GP registrars and older, more experienced GPs. This is often linked to frustration with the current systems of paperwork, and perceived conflict between the role of patient advocate and assessment of fitness for work.

Research

During the last 10 years of the growth of research and development in primary care, a useful evidence base has begun to emerge from research into sickness certification conducted in Scandinavia, the UK (Mersey Primary Care Consortium) and the rest of Europe under the umbrella of the European Public Health Association. In the UK, recent joint Department of Health and Department for Work and Pensions welfare reforms such as the Job Retention and Rehabilitation pilot and the 'Pathways to Work' Condition Management Programme (CMP) pilot have led to the development of a variety of interventions that are accessible from primary care.

Programmes

GP responses to these programmes have generally been very favourable, as the programmes offer help to patients who have been previously problematic – for example, middle-aged men with musculoskeletal problems who are getting too old for heavy manual jobs, but who do not have educational qualifications or transferable skills. In these cases, joint initiatives with rehabilitation and Jobcentre Plus partners can transfer the patient from a medical model into the social and educational arenas where they rightly belong. An awareness-raising project for Lancashire CMP found that 70% of local GPs expressed a positive interest in rehabilitation/certification issues, with a third of these wishing to take a more active part in the pilot, such as hosting a Jobcentre Plus adviser in their practice.

Initiatives

Other recent initiatives relating to access to cognitive–behavioural therapy (CBT), including the availability of graduate mental health workers and computerised CBT (compare this with the National Institute for Clinical Excellence (NICE) guidelines for management of depression), and the launch of the Expert Patient Programme (EPP) as a social enterprise, mean that GPs finally have access to a range of appropriate interventions to help their patients to cope with chronic disabling conditions and to regain economic independence whenever possible. As yet, this aspect of the management of long-term conditions does not have the high profile of the arguably more disabling and medicalising approaches to monitoring and prescribing that are currently part of the Quality and Outcomes Framework (QOF) governing GP remuneration. However, there is a strong possibility that occupational issues/ sickness certification may be included in the future, and NICE is currently developing guidelines for long-term conditions and incapacity.

Although it has been shown that unemployed people visit their doctor more frequently than those who are employed, there is not yet any convincing evidence that programmes such as CMP or EPP directly reduce consultation and/or prescribing rates. This is probably because this type of programme promotes health literacy and enables better use of medication and services, including both encouraging self-care and increasing appropriate help-seeking for those who had previously given up hope of medical help, which obviously tend to cancel each other out in consultation rate statistics. Thus there are clear ways of making the GP management of incapacity more productive and less frustrating, while not necessarily reducing the overall workload.

GP approaches to sickness certification

Research into GP attitudes conducted by Julia Hiscock for the Department for Work and Pensions described the main ways in which GPs approach sickness certification.[1] These include a variety of beliefs, ranging from the idea that certification is a statutory duty which should not be the responsibility of GPs at all, to the concept of sickness certification as a therapeutic intervention in a holistic care package. Some GPs also felt uncertain about their capacity to assess fitness for work, and felt that they needed more training. Further research has been carried out by Debbie Cohen at Cardiff University, leading to the development of a training package for GPs.

The Department for Work and Pensions has, over the years, developed a number of training packs and desk aids to support GPs in certification issues, and these can be accessed at www.dwp.gov.uk/medical. This website also includes useful information on Benefits Agency processes, different types of sick notes (e.g. Med 3, 4 and 5 forms), and the Personal Capability Assessment (PCA), which generally takes place after the patient becomes eligible for Incapacity Benefit (around 28 weeks off sick). Some GPs feel that independent medical assessment should ideally take place as early as possible in order to allow the GP to concentrate on treating the patient rather than on their fitness for work. The results of the PCA are now passed on to GPs, which makes continuing management easier in primary care.

Incapacitating health professionals

Unfortunately, the behaviour of health professionals in general, but particularly those involved in sickness certification, may be a major barrier to their patients' rehabilitation for work. This includes labelling or stigmatising patients (e.g. 'no-good bum', 'timewaster', 'heartsink patient') and thereby damaging the doctor–patient partnership, and/or excessive illness validation as through paternalistic chronic disease management protocols and/or over-investigation. Loss of confidence leads to either passive dependence or alienation of the patient and prolonged incapacity.

Common traps in certification practice

There are four common traps for the certifying doctor, each of which can be caricatured as a type of bird – the pigeon, the hen, the hawk and the dove – representing common attitudes to sickness certification. These approaches are apparently reasonable in themselves, but will affect a patient's recovery and return to work in different ways, leading to potentially adverse consequences for the patient, the doctor, the employer and Jobcentre Plus. This is easily demonstrated by applying the four approaches to a hypothetical incapacity case.

The following is a 'typical' sick-note request:

A 45-year-old man who has worked as a bricklayer for 25 years suffering from severe low back pain. Previous episodes of increasing frequency and duration over the last five years.

The pigeon

The pigeon feels that sickness certification is 'not my pigeon – I am here to treat the patient, and it is up to Jobcentre Plus to assess fitness for work.' Pigeon doctors view a request for a sick note as a 'quickie' consultation which gives them time to catch up time during a busy surgery. They often have large lists and carry a high workload, working in a very transactional way to get through large numbers of patients in a relatively short time. This may have the following consequences for the doctor, the patient, the employer and Jobcentre Plus:

 › Doctor: likely to give a short sick note for 1 to 2 weeks, with analgesics/ non-steroidal anti-inflammatory drugs (NSAIDs) initially. If the patient does not recover, the doctor will give certificates of increasing duration and repeat prescriptions for painkillers, often without reviewing the patient personally, and refer them on to other services (e.g. physiotherapy). Responds in an ad-hoc way (with irritation) to further bureaucracy from Jobcentre Plus, such as requests for a Med 4 certificate for Incapacity Benefit or IB113/factual reports.
 › Patient: increasingly despondent about continuing pain and incapacity, eventually leading to secondary depression, job loss due to prolonged sickness absence, and long-term Incapacity Benefit claim. Increasing demands on the health service, such as referrals to secondary care, musculoskeletal services, pain management, etc., often with long waiting times which further delay recovery.
 › Employer: uncertainty over prognosis due to lack of information on sick notes, leading to difficulties in covering the job, economic losses and eventual sacking of the employee.
 › Jobcentre Plus: increased bureaucracy involved in following up minimal information on certificates. Long-term Incapacity Benefit costs.

The dove

Doves are friendly and obliging, popular with patients and colleagues alike, but their gentle 'cooing' disguises a clear grasp of the importance of boundaries. Doves may prefer to take a salaried position, and may combine this with other sessional work or family responsibilities.

- **Doctor:** will ask the patient how long he needs off work and write his certificates accordingly, on the grounds that the patient himself is best placed to assess whether he can do his job or not. The dove is supportive, issuing repeat prescriptions for strong painkillers to ease the patient's suffering, and will refer the patient on to other services according to their level of anxiety and frequency of attendance.
- **Patient:** initially grateful to his supportive doctor, but after some time begins to feel frustrated by the lack of progress. Job loss and continuing pain result in low mood and feelings of helplessness, compounded by drowsiness from excessive use of analgesics. The patient may become a frequent attender, constantly seeking further interventions, 'second opinions' and the like, in the vain hope of reclaiming his life.
- **Employer:** receives rapid responses to queries concerning prognosis, etc., confirming what the patient has reported already. Job loss will occur after a variable period, according to the patient's terms and conditions of employment and how quickly he gives up hope of being able to go back to work.
- **Jobcentre Plus:** satisfied by the dove's capacity to complete and return certificates and reports on time. The resulting Incapacity Benefit claim may be upheld or overturned at the PCA (according to the approach of the examining doctor), but long-term events will be largely independent of the dove's input.

The hawk

The hawk feels a duty to protect the taxpayer from the 'work-shy skiver.' Hawks often work in areas of high social deprivation with high rates of unemployment and Incapacity Benefit claims (medicalised unemployment). They may be single-handed GPs with a high level of control over their practices, and fed up with what they perceive to be people cheating the system.

- **Doctor:** likely to contest the requests for continuing sickness certification, quoting guidelines about physical exercise being good for simple back pain. This may result in repeated short sickness absences due to recurrent back pain provoked by manual labour, and consequent job loss due to the patient's poor sickness record.
- **Patient:** angry with the hawk for not taking his pain seriously. This may result in aggressive help-seeking behaviour, inappropriate visits to out-of-hours services and Accident and Emergency departments, and visits to other GPs who may be more sympathetic to his cause (thus undermining

the authority of the hawk). Depression and frustration are expressed as anger and aggression, thus inhibiting others from providing help and support. The patient's back condition may be aggravated by continuing exposure to heavy lifting, etc.

> **Employer:** frustration with continuing situation of employee, who is seen as unfit for his job and unreliable. Colleagues may resent having to take on his share of the heavy/unpleasant aspects of the job. Breakdown of work relationships resulting in job loss.

> **Jobcentre Plus:** presented with client who is difficult to manage and aggressive, and who may enter into further acrimonious relationships with staff, possibly resulting in his failing a PCA and transfer to Jobseeker's Allowance, with minimal support for finding alternative employment.

The hen

The hen feels a duty to defend the patient against the 'wicked system' which pressurises people who are 'genuinely sick' to go back to work. The patient needs to be protected from work which has damaged him, and is entitled to draw on the system into which he has paid for 25 years.

> **Doctor:** likely to be sympathetic to the patient's plight, investigating his back pain and discovering that he has osteoarthritis of his lumbar spine. Explains that the patient's job has caused wear and tear, and that he will probably 'never be able to work again.' Refers the patient for physiotherapy, and if this is not beneficial will refer him on for pain management. The hen gives relatively long-duration sick notes with explanations to the employer and Jobcentre Plus, leading quickly to job loss and long-term incapacity. Rapidly diagnoses and treats secondary depression.

> **Patient:** shocked to hear his diagnosis and resentful of the way his job has caused him to become prematurely old. Rapid job loss, depression and dependence on Incapacity Benefit, but grateful to supportive doctor. May lead to chronic illness behaviour with adaptation to economic dependence, secondary gain and alternative lifestyles.

> **Employer:** rapidly informed about the patient's poor prognosis, leading to early sacking of employee with minimal economic loss to company.

> **Jobcentre Plus:** long-term Incapacity Benefit claim, possibly contested at the PCA, followed by appeal and re-instigation of a claim for 'genuine incapacity.'

Most GPs will recognise a little of themselves in the pigeon, the dove, the hawk and/or the hen, but most of us will not have had the time or the opportunity to reflect on the sometimes far-reaching outcomes of these caricatured approaches to sickness certification. Later in this chapter we hope to show how each of the birds can refashion their approach to improve outcomes for themselves, their patients, their employers, and even Jobcentre Plus and the taxpayer.

Sick-note diagnoses

Much to the despair of individuals and organisations (such as the Department for Work and Pensions) who work with classifications and codes and scientific diagnoses, GPs continue to write on sick notes the description of the cause of sickness absence which they and their patient have agreed upon. This may not be a medical diagnosis at all (e.g. 'stress'), and may or may not have indicators of attribution as well as causation (e.g. 'bereavement'). A sick note is intended to be seen by a variety of people who may have differing perspectives on the patient's incapacity, including the patient him- or herself, the employer/ line manager, human resources personnel, occupational health professionals, Jobcentre Plus employees, Benefits Agency adjudicators and independent medical advisers at the PCA. Trying to keep all of these people happy may considerably constrain what a GP actually writes.

   Many GPs do not realise that Jobcentre Plus has a comprehensive list of conditions and the expected duration of absence for these, to which their adjudicators can refer. This means, for example, that a 6-month duration of absence following hysterectomy is likely to be questioned. In this case, the unduly prolonged absence may be due to the patient becoming depressed by a perceived loss of femininity, and the reason for absence has thus subtly changed and could more accurately be described as secondary depression.

Changing diagnosis

Recognising that the actual cause of absence has changed may be of paramount importance if such a patient is to be helped to recover and return to work. This requires a range of possible interventions from the GP, including acknowledgement and/or discussion of the underlying emotional issues, counselling or cognitive–behavioural therapy and/or antidepressant medication as appropriate. Loss of confidence and/or depression is a very common barrier to return to work, regardless of the initial diagnosis, and this was confirmed in the Merseyside study of GP certification, which showed that the most common secondary diagnosis was depression.

Mild or moderate mental health problems are now the most common cause of incapacity for work overall in the UK, and are responsible for more days off work than any other condition.[2] Other European countries still quote musculoskeletal disorders/back pain as top of the list, but this may be due to cultural differences in labelling rather than actual prevalence of disease. It is known that men, particularly those in physically demanding jobs with a masculine culture, tend to present with physical rather than emotional pain, and that in recent years, in our post-industrial society, 'diagnoses' such as 'stress' have become much more socially acceptable.

The prevalence of different 'diagnoses' on GP sick notes of increasing duration of incapacity is shown in Figure 4.1. This highlights the crucial nature of mental health problems as a cause of incapacity of longer duration, with all the associated risks to the patient of long-term benefit dependence.

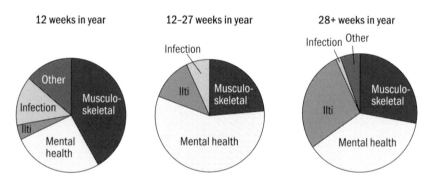

Figure 4.1 Epidemiology of sick-note diagnoses related to duration of incapacity. *Source:* Mersey Primary Care R&D Consortium.

Work in the Mersey Primary Care Consortium also demonstrates a difference in the mean duration of time off work related to whether or not the certifying GP attributes the mental health problem to an external cause. Certificates for stress and bereavement are significantly shorter than those for 'pure' anxiety and depression, and those associated with alcohol and drug abuse are the longest of all. This probably means that many GPs, whether consciously or not, recognise the difference between symptoms which have a temporary social cause, those which indicate a mental disorder per se, and those which are connected with longer-term aberrant behaviour or personality problems. Clearly the management of these conditions should be different, and the Benefits Agency would be wise to pick up clues from GPs rather than asking for 'diagnostic codes.'

Attribution

As mentioned previously in relation to length of sickness absence, the perceived cause of the illness may influence the duration of incapacity for work. In the case of workplace stress (which may be presented as a 'diagnosis'), validated time off work may play a significant role in the patient's recovery, and returning too soon or into a dysfunctional or conflict-ridden workplace may further aggravate the illness.

Stress inside the workplace

Liaison with the patient's employer, human resources officer, line manager and/or occupational health professional may be very helpful in this situation, although by the time the stress of workplace bullying, difficult working relationships or unwelcome changes in the content or circumstances of employment has resulted in mental health problems and incapacity for work, the best option for the patient is often a change of employment. Personal advisers or the Disability Employment Adviser at Jobcentre Plus can assist in this situation.

Stress outside the workplace

When symptoms are caused by stress in the home, family illness, marital (or other relationship) conflict or divorce, an early return to work may aid the patient's recovery from anxiety- or depression-related illness by removing the patient from the stressful situation and distracting them from what may be relatively insoluble problems. Again, liaison with a sympathetic employer may keep the patient at work, with resulting benefits for both employer and employee.

Social stressors

A social attribution may necessitate a social intervention if the patient is to recover (e.g. relationship or debt counselling necessitating referral to the voluntary sector, such as the Citizens Advice Bureau, welfare rights organisations or Relate, or to a counselling service either attached to or external to the practice). When referring a patient to an outside agency, care should be taken to ensure that the staff are appropriately qualified and the organisation is reputable and accountable.

Biomedical attribution

A biomedical attribution for sickness absence causation, such as back injury or clinical depression, may make the GP feel more comfortable, but frequently causes longer periods of incapacity awaiting investigations, surgery or compensation, while the patient adopts a sick role validated by the doctor and/or external agencies or specialists. All too often the underlying barriers to rehabilitation for work are psychosocial rather than physical, and the patient will not recover until these are addressed or resolve spontaneously.

The longest periods of incapacity may be associated with serious/terminal illnesses (in which circumstances a limited amount of work may be therapeutic in maintaining the patient's sense of identity and usefulness, but advice concerning occupational health and safety may be necessary) and substance abuse (in which some kinds of employment are unsuitable or dangerous, and specialist intervention is often required).

Models of incapacity

As was mentioned in Chapter 1, incapacity may be interpreted within either a medical or a social model, and both have much to offer (*see* Figure 4.2).

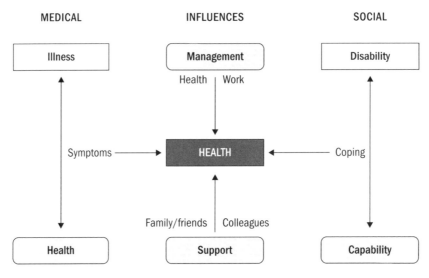

Figure 4.2 Influences on work capability.

THE MEDICAL MODEL OF REHABILITATION FOR WORK

Using a traditional medical model of illness and health, conventional management is to make a diagnosis and initiate treatment, often appropriate medication regimes, and/or refer the patient for specialist advice. When considering rehabilitation for work, the most pressing consideration may not be the disease/diagnosis, but the symptoms that the patient is currently experiencing and their potential amelioration. Vocational rehabilitation requires that the patient is able to carry out their work regardless of whether their disease can be or has been cured. This functional approach is similar to consideration of Activities of Daily Living for a stroke victim by an occupational therapist, and has resulted in occupational therapists playing a key role in Condition Management Programmes.

GPs are accustomed to working in the mode of symptom management, as shown by the frequency of symptom codes in the Read coding system, which was developed specifically for general practice. Indeed, during the transition to paper-free working, many GPs were uncomfortable with the perceived need for a consultation 'diagnosis' on computer. For most people visiting their GP, a major consideration is the search for relief from troublesome symptoms.

As was mentioned in Chapter 1, it is possible for an individual to continue working despite suffering from a serious or potentially fatal disease, provided that the symptoms are controlled. Conversely, it may be impossible to work if the symptoms are severe, however trivial the disease may be.

Symptoms of mental ill health

The most important of these symptoms for rehabilitation for work in primary care are anxiety and depression, as they are very common compared with more serious and psychotic symptoms such as hallucinations, delusions and major thought disorder, which generally require specialist help before a return to work can be considered.

Anxiety in itself has no direct relationship with duration of sickness absence, as it may have confounding effects. For example, a patient may return quickly from sickness absence due to increased problem-solving activity triggered by anxiety, or their return may be delayed by the depression which is frequently associated with clinical anxiety.[3]

Depression is the most common barrier to return to work, due to loss of confidence, low self-esteem, poor memory and concentration, and sleep disturbance, all of which are associated symptoms. Even sub-clinical depressive disorders and ordinary distress associated with life events can have a relatively major effect on a person's ability to return to work. Regardless of the initial 'diagnosis' or reason for going off sick, return to work is directly related to the number of symptoms of depression that a person is experiencing. In the current system, which rewards GPs for recording a diagnosis of depression, matched with a measure of severity, doctors have an obvious aid to predicting barriers to return to work associated with depressive symptoms, and a prompt for taking suitable action.

The place of cognitive–behavioural therapy

NICE guidelines on the treatment of depression recommend the use of anti-depressant medication and cognitive–behavioural therapy (CBT), including computerised CBT. Both of these interventions are known to be effective in treating the symptoms of depression, although patient engagement and compliance may be very problematic. Only 30% of those referred for a mental health intervention are likely to turn up for even the first appointment, with probably similar rates of compliance with medication. Potential solutions to this problem are further explored in the section on the social model of rehabilitation for work (see below).

A systematic review by the British Occupational Health Research Foundation of workplace interventions for people with common mental problems[4] found that the only intervention which is proven to improve rates of return to work is CBT. Although antidepressant medication may relieve the symptoms of depression, it may be some time after symptom resolution before the patient returns to work.[5] The Layard recommendations[6] concerning CBT in primary care, and the NICE guidelines recommending computerised CBT, which is already being piloted in primary care and is likely to become more widely available in the near future, mean that most GPs will soon have access to CBT for patients who need it. If used appropriately, this should have a markedly beneficial effect on rehabilitation for work in primary care.

Symptoms of physical ill health

The most important of these are pain, immobility, breathlessness and fatigue. Useful interventions to control these symptoms include suitable medication and exercise. Prescription of drugs still tends to be associated with the power and status of doctors, although other healthcare professionals (e.g. nurse practitioners) now have a small but increasingly significant role. For GPs, giving a prescription may also be a way of bringing a difficult consultation to an end, or part of a transactional approach to doctor–patient relationships which avoids tackling the deeper psychosocial issues. However, patient education concerning appropriate use of medication, potential side-effects, etc., is often lacking.

Pain

Most patients with chronic pain will have access to analgesics but may not understand how best to use them. For example, they may be drowsy during the day due to the over-use of opiates, but toss and turn all night when the effect of their short-acting analgesics has worn off. A patient who understands their treatment is more likely to use it effectively, and is enabled to self-care, with a consequent reduction in (ineffective) service use.[7] The smallest amount of the safest available medicine is usually the best choice when managing long-term conditions, and side-effects may sometimes be useful (e.g. drowsiness at night).

Educational interventions concerning medication use, as provided in Pain Management Programmes and Condition Management Programmes, show measurable beneficial effects on patient perceptions of relief from medications using tools such as the Brief Pain Inventory. This type of educational intervention can easily be administered by a nurse or allied health professional with appropriate training (*see* Table 4.1).

The biopsychosocial approach adopted by mainstream NHS pain management programmes has proven beneficial effects on the levels of pain experienced and on how patients cope with their pain. Expanding the social components of such interventions through partnership working with Jobcentre Plus, occupational health departments and employers can make this type of approach very much more successful in improving both health outcomes and working ability.

Immobility and fatigue

This may be linked with pain, musculoskeletal conditions and/or obesity, and is best managed by graded exercise, which can usefully be accessed through Local Authority Exercise on Referral initiatives, with physiotherapy advice and treatment where necessary. Advice on pacing is very important for these patients, as they tend to become trapped in a vicious circle of over-activity and collapse, which exacerbates their symptoms. This advice can be given in the form of a leaflet with guidance from a GP or nurse, which can also be applicable to symptoms of fatigue or tiredness, including those associated with myalgic encephalopathy (ME)/chronic fatigue syndrome.

Breathlessness

Management includes treatment of the underlying cause (e.g. correct use of asthma inhalers, heart failure medication, weight reduction programmes and graded exercise, as above). Specialist referral may be necessary for further investigation of the cause and/or advice on optimal management, particularly in the case of major heart, lung and neurological disease. However, waiting for investigations is frequently cited as a (spurious) cause of sickness absence. If symptoms are adequately controlled, most patients are better off at work than sitting at home worrying about the possible diagnosis or prognosis.

Table 4.1 Explaining analgesics to patients[8]

	NAMES	INDICATION	EFFECTS	SIDE-EFFECTS	AVAILABILITY	TIPS
Painkillers	Paracetamol	Day-to-day pain, any cause Fever	Mild to moderate painkiller	Overdose harms liver and kidneys, and may be fatal (2 weeks afterwards)	Over the counter in limited quantities	Very safe up to 8 tablets a day. Can be used in pregnancy
Anti-inflammatory drugs	Aspirin, ibuprofen, other non-steroidal anti-inflammatory drugs (NSAIDs), COX inhibitors	Pain, fever and inflammation/ swelling (e.g. arthritis)	Immediate painkiller and increasing anti-inflammatory effect	Stomach irritation, heartburn, ulcers, bleeding/ haemorrhage (bleeding can be fatal). Asthma/ wheeze	Over the counter: aspirin, Nurofen, Cuprofen, Brufen, Prescription only: diclofenac/ Voltarol, Lederfen, etc.	Not safe if you have a bad stomach, always take after food, better taken regularly for several days to allow anti-inflammatory effects to manifest
'Euphoriants'	Codeine (including combinations with paracetamol, e.g. co-codamol), dihydrocodeine (DHC), tramadol, controlled drugs (e.g. morphine)	More severe pain	Moderate painkiller and mild euphoriant	Constipation (advise increased fibre intake, e.g. Weetabix, and fluids), nausea, drowsiness	Over the counter: milder, e.g. 8 mg codeine with paracetamol (co-codamol); stronger, e.g. 30 mg codeine Prescription only: e.g. Kapake	Useful at night when drowsiness is an advantage, particularly sustained-release preparations (e.g. tramadol), as effects last all night

The *medical model* of symptom management in the context of rehabilitation for work therefore depends on a three-pronged approach:

1 appropriate therapy
2 patient education
3 graded activity.

THE SOCIAL MODEL OF REHABILITATION FOR WORK

Having considered above what symptoms a patient experiences and how they can be managed in a health-promoting fashion, the social model (*see* Figure 4.2) considers disability and capability, and the coping strategies which might influence the balance between incapacity and recovery. Defining recovery in this context is more about what a person can do in spite of (or even because of) their disease/disability. This is expressed very clearly in an old Viking poem:

HAVAMAL: (THE SAYINGS OF THE VIKINGS)

Everyone has his use:

The lame rides a horse,　　　　　*(in spite of disability, i.e. extra speed on horseback)*

The maimed drives the herd,　　　*(in spite of disability, i.e. slower-paced task)*

The deaf is brave in battle.　　　*(because of disability, i.e. not frightened by noise)*

A man is better blind than buried.　*(see line 1)*

A dead man is deft at nothing.　　*(only death takes away all usefulness)*

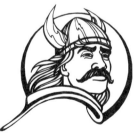

This must be one of the earliest examples of reasonable adjustments!

Coping strategies which facilitate return to work

The way that a patient copes with disability (functional impairment) depends on their own preferred coping styles and on societal influences (e.g. family, colleagues, etc.). It has been suggested in the past that individual preferred coping styles are relatively fixed, and that they are directly related to personality. However, research on the influence of coping styles on return to work[8] identified a pattern associated with rehabilitation for work which can be facilitated by contact with health professionals and by Condition Management Programmes.

The *social model* of rehabilitation for work after a period of illness depends on enhancing the patient's ability to cope with their condition by:

1 acceptance – acknowledgement of their limitations
2 positive reframing – looking for alternatives
3 planning for the future.

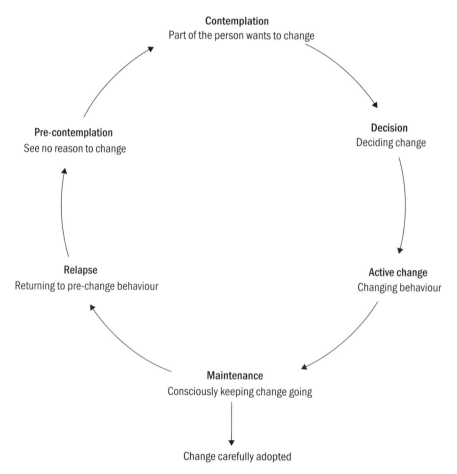

Figure 4.3 The cycle of change.

Evaluation of Lancashire CMP has shown that participation in the programme results in increased use of these coping styles (as measured by the Brief COPE) and return to work, even after long periods of incapacity. This is presumably linked with the CBT-based approach of the CMP, designed to move the individual participant through the cycle of change (*see* Figure 4.3) and to promote patient empowerment.

Within a one-to-one therapeutic relationship, as in primary care, the acknowledged technique for empowering a patient to make health-promoting changes is known as 'motivational interviewing.' This technique is widely taught in nursing and undergraduate medical courses, but those of us who qualified more than 10 years ago are unlikely to have had the advantage of formal teaching on the subject.

Motivational interviewing

This is a brief psychotherapeutic intervention, based on the principles of motivational psychology, which is designed to initiate and support the process of behaviour change. The technique was developed in recognition of the fact that patients are unlikely to change their health-related behaviours, comply with treatment regimens, etc., unless they are motivated to do so, and that traditional paternalistic ways of imparting information do not necessarily motivate the patient to act on this information.

In brief, motivational interviewing involves assessing the patient's readiness to change by ascertaining the following:

1   What stage is the patient in now? (*see* Figure 4.3)
2   What are the barriers to change?
3   What are the drivers for change?
4   What information does the patient need in order to change?
5   How should this information be given?

The course of action/treatment plan can then be negotiated between the health professional and the patient, with proven beneficial effects on the likelihood of the patient carrying out the agreed plan. Adopting this approach in the context of rehabilitation for work/sickness certification is clearly useful, as it enables the GP to influence the patient to identify and accept their limitations, reframe the possibilities and move on (*see* section on coping strategies above). The aim of motivational interviewing in this context is to enable the patient to cope better with their condition by facilitating self-care, thereby enhancing work capability.

Improving the management of incapacity

In order to appropriately manage a consultation about incapacity for work, a biopsychosocial approach (i.e. assessment of the physical, psychological and social factors involved in the patient's decision to be absent from work) is vital. Research for Merseyside Health Action Zone (HAZ) into the barriers to and facilitators of return to work following mental health problems[9] suggests that the most successful professional approach involves a friendly and supportive doctor who:

1 adopts a personal rather than a procedural approach
2 establishes a decision-making partnership with the patient
3 arranges timely and appropriate expert referral.

Table 4.2 demonstrates the relationship between professional consultation skills which lead to optimal management of the patient's symptoms, and enhancement of the patient's coping abilities.

Table 4.2 Optimal management of the incapacity consultation

	CONSULTATION SKILLS	SYMPTOM MANAGEMENT	COPING STRATEGIES
1	Biopsychosocial assessment	Appropriate therapy	Acceptance
2	Motivational interviewing	Patient education	Positive reframing
3	Decision-making partnership	Graded activity	Planning

A detailed and practical breakdown of this approach as it applies to the health professional can be found in the Appendix (*see* page 181).

Revisiting the 'typical' sick-note request

Returning to the bird model, we can re-examine how our pigeon, dove, hawk and hen might respond to the same 45-year-old patient with simple back pain and a manual job, having read this chapter and reflected on their own practice. In order to do this, it is not necessary to radically change the practice of a lifetime, as most GPs are aware that there are always a number of different routes leading to a positive outcome.

The pigeon

The pigeon's main strength is decisiveness. Pigeons have an ability to come to conclusions and take action very quickly, associated with brevity of communication. As we have seen, this can lead to increased levels of bureaucracy and repeated patient demands for certificates, reports and referrals. The pigeon's skill in rapid decision making can be remodelled to include early recognition that this patient's problem is basically about being too old for his physically demanding job. This realisation may radically alter the consequences for doctor, patient, employer and Jobcentre Plus.

> **Doctor:** writes a sick note for back pain, commenting in the 'Remarks' section that the patient is unfit for heavy lifting, thus alerting the employer and Jobcentre Plus to the likelihood that the patient will not be able to continue in his present job. Also warns the patient that he will need to change his job if his back continues to trouble him. When asked for a Med 4 form for an Incapacity Benefit claim, fills in 'low back pain with secondary depression' and suggests that the patient could be fit in future for a job that involves no heavy lifting. Reduced demand for bureaucracy, due to earlier clarity of certification, results in more time available to treat the patient (e.g. by referral to Jobcentre Plus for further help and advice, including Condition Management Programme, if available).

> **Patient:** may be eligible under the Disability Discrimination Act for workplace adjustments if his condition has affected him for a year or more. Unlikely to find light work on a building site, so may still lose his current job, but will then be eligible for help with retraining while claiming Incapacity Benefit. More aware of the prognosis from an earlier stage, so will be initially despondent, but more likely to obtain help to move on. Following retraining is likely to be re-employed in a more suitable job for the next 20 years, rather than claiming benefits.

> **Employer:** clarity of certification means that a decision to change the job description or end the contract can be made more quickly and easily, thus avoiding economic losses.

> **Jobcentre Plus:** efforts can be directed towards helping the individual to retrain and find suitable employment, instead of chasing up the doctor for further reports.

The dove

The dove's main strength is an awareness of boundaries, which early on enables them to realise that the main problem relates to the patient's employment rather than a medical condition per se. This leads to sickness certification which makes it clear that the patient is unfit for their current work.

> **Doctor:** gives a sick note indicating that the patient is not likely to be fit for work for some time. The dove treats the back pain by giving the patient a handout on the management of simple back pain, with

education on optimal use of medications to maximise night-time sleep and daytime alertness, while making it clear that the solution to the problem lies in the work arena rather than the medical one. Refers the patient on to a Condition Management Programme (if available) as soon as they lose their job and claim Incapacity Benefit. This involves more work in the short term, but minimises the patient's demands in the longer term.

- **Patient:** clear at an early stage that the best way forward will be through employment options, and less likely to become depressed as a result of inaction and helplessness. If solutions are delayed, or he is angry about the inevitable job loss, he is more likely to vent his frustration on his employer or Jobcentre Plus than on his doctor!
- **Employer:** gets the message that the patient is unlikely to be fit for his current job with a minimum of delay, and responds accordingly.
- **Jobcentre Plus:** able to move forward quickly on to Condition Management Programme and retraining options, thus minimising the patient's time on Incapacity Benefit and rapidly helping him to regain his independence.

The hawk

The hawk's main strength is in assessment. It is the hawk who initially realised that this patient is not actually unfit to work for his living, but because he failed to take account of the psychosocial aspects of assessment, this did not lead to a beneficial outcome. If the hawk can work with the patient to plan for his future, the outcomes will be less painful for all of the stakeholders.

- **Doctor:** a sick note stating 'Fit for work' but including under Remarks 'No heavy lifting' is likely to lead to rapid job loss for the patient. The patient is less likely to be angry with the doctor, particularly if the hawk has explained his conclusions that the back pain will settle down provided that the patient has the right treatment, keeps active, and seeks a less physically demanding job.
- **Patient:** provided that the hawk assesses him thoroughly initially, is likely to feel that he has a champion to defend his rights, and may be motivated enough to find a new job himself without recourse to benefits claims. Very much reduced levels of help-seeking from the NHS, but may be militant in demanding his employment rights (e.g. under the Disability Discrimination Act).
- **Employer:** may be angry with the doctor rather than with the patient, as the company is put under pressure to find less physically demanding

work. Reduced likelihood of economic losses and lower levels of frustration overall.

❯ **Jobcentre Plus:** may not come into contact with the patient if he manages to find himself alternative employment. If he claims Jobseeker's Allowance or Incapacity Benefit following job loss, he is less likely to be aggressive, more ready for retraining, etc.

The hen

The hen's main strength is an empathic relationship with the patient. This means that a friendly and supportive consultation style comes naturally, and once the hen has explored the barriers to work and discovered that the main problem is the physically demanding nature of the job combined with ageing, they will negotiate with the patient's employer and Jobcentre Plus as necessary to help the patient towards more suitable work. This can be done while managing the patient's symptoms as before.

❯ **Doctor:** awareness of the wider picture will enable the hen to be more proactive in communicating with the employer (by letter, telephone or by further information on the sick note), and in managing the patient's symptoms by motivational interviewing. This will lead to a more satisfying outcome for all, including the doctor.

❯ **Patient:** normalises his back problem rather than catastrophising it. Will continue to be grateful to his doctor, but will be less dependent and more empowered to make changes in his life and work. With this level of support, his back pain is likely to improve quite quickly, and his length of time on benefits will be short.

❯ **Employer:** in these circumstances may be able to find alternative work for the patient, but if this is impossible, has sufficient information to act appropriately to prevent undue economic losses.

❯ **Jobcentre Plus:** may have little contact with the patient, unless he loses his job, in which case the Incapacity Benefit Personal Advisers will be able to work with the doctor to move the patient into more appropriate work.

CONCLUSIONS

By recognising the biopsychosocial nature of sickness certification, the doctor can make appropriate use of therapeutic and communication skills to maximise the management of symptoms, enhance the patient's coping strategies, and improve liaison with outside agencies, in order to facilitate rehabilitation for work.

REFERENCES

1 Hiscock J, Hodgson P, Peters S, Westlake D, Gabbay M. *Engaging Physicians, Benefiting Patients: a qualitative study.* Research Report 256. London: Department for Work and Pensions; 2005.

2 Shiels C, Gabbay M, Ford FM. Patient factors associated with duration of certified sickness absence and transition to long-term incapacity. *Br J Gen Pract.* 2004; **54**(499): 86–91.

3 Wanberg C. Antecedents and outcomes of coping behaviours among unemployed and re-employed individuals. *J Applied Psychol.* 1997; **82**(5): 731–44.

4 British Occupational Health Research Foundation. *Workplace Interventions for People with Common Mental Health Problems: evidence review and recommendations.* London: BOHRF; September 2005. www.bohrf.org.uk/downloads/cmh_rev.pdf

5 Mintz J, Mintz LI, Arruda MJ, Hwang SS. Treatments of depression and the functional capacity to work. *Arch Gen Psychiatry.* 1992; **49**(10): 761–8.

6 The Centre for Economic Performance's Policy Group. *The Depression Report: a new deal for depression and anxiety disorders.* London: London School of Economics; June 2006.

7 Carder PC, Vuckovic N, Green CA. Negotiating medications: patient perceptions of long-term medication use. *J Clin Pharm Ther.* 2003; **28**(5): 409–17.

8 Ford F. *Making the Most of Medicines.* Lancashire Condition Management Programme; 2006.

9 Ford F, Canvin K. *What can health professionals do to promote the functional recovery of people with mental health problems?* Annual Scientific Conference, Society of Academic Primary Care; July 2003.

CHAPTER 5

Perspective of a lay adviser in occupational health

It is widely believed that early intervention to prevent prolonged sickness absence is best. This view is based perhaps on the observation that it is very difficult to help people back to work – even if they want to go back – when they have been off sick for months. However, the arguments against early intervention are also strong. Most spells of sickness absence are self-limiting, and investigating and intervening in each one would be impossible to justify in terms of cost-effectiveness, as well as being logistically difficult.

In practice, early intervention is rarely achieved. In the following sections I shall discuss the help needed during the period leading up to sickness absence and at various stages thereafter, and where help can be obtained. A second theme will be the need for methods of deciding who needs help at each stage.

The kinds of help needed are diverse, but also poorly integrated and far from uniformly available to all, so this chapter will also consider unmet needs and how they might be met. In the final section, particular attention is paid to one of the unsolved problems for return-to-work services, namely how to help people with mental health problems to return to and stay in work. I shall look at events from the patient's perspective, using my experience as a non-medical occupational health adviser in primary healthcare, helping people who are referred to me by their GP.

UNSTABLE WORK: POTENTIAL FOR PREVENTION

Before a patient takes time off from work, there is often a period characterised by physical pain or acute psychological symptoms accompanied by uncertainty and anxiety about work. This state has been described by Anne Chamberlain and colleagues at the University of Leeds as *work instability*, when the requirements of the job can be fulfilled – just – but often with help from understanding work colleagues, or against the advice of the individual's partner or their GP. An observant manager may be aware that something is wrong, and a health surveillance system at work might detect a risk of worsening health. For the most part, however, when employees are struggling to carry out their jobs they do their best to disguise the fact. The experiences of sickness-related redundancy and dismissal in the 1980s and early 1990s remain in the collective memory of the workforce.

This is the earliest stage at which the ability to work is limited by a health problem. I shall use the term *work limitation* rather than 'absence from work' as the criterion for action, as there is plenty of evidence to suggest that merely avoiding sickness absence in the short term, sometimes described as *presenteeism*, is no guarantee of fitness in the longer term. Work limitation may also be the maturing of a chronic or progressive health problem that, with sensitive management of job design, could be accommodated without causing a crisis.

What can be done at this stage? Now is the time for planning. A breakdown in physical health is common as workers – particularly those in manual trades – get older. Planning ahead means recognising this situation, and then introducing and evaluating options. Age discrimination legislation and the need to include older workers in the workforce should lead to the use of early screening to redesign work so that it is conducive to longer working lives, an approach that has been strongly promoted in other parts of Europe.

The *Finnish Work Ability Index* is a simple 7-component screening tool for identifying people who are at risk of leaving work prematurely. Like the *Work Instability Scale* that emerged from Chamberlain's work, it has been designed for use when people are still at work, and can be utilised as a part of routine surveillance by occupational health staff. The seven components (see below) found to be useful for predicting early retirement are immediately accessible to GPs either as a matter of record (sickness absence, current diseases, mental resources), or by asking the patient directly.

SEVEN COMPONENTS OF THE FINNISH WORK ABILITY INDEX

Current work ability compared with lifetime best

Work ability in relation to the demands of the job.

Number of current diseases diagnosed by a physician

Estimated work impairment due to diseases

Sick leave during the past year

Own estimation of work ability 2 years from now

Mental resources (in relation to work and non-work activities)

To prevent this time of 'unstable work' becoming the prelude to a period of time off sick, the worker/patient needs the following:

> *line management* to take a flexible approach to work limitation, have good communication skills, and have good relationships with occupational health staff

> *work colleagues* to have good relationships with other staff, whose relationship with line managers is based on trust

> *occupational health staff* to be mandated to carry out primary prevention, not merely sickness absence interventions

> *general practitioners* to have time to ask about work limitation in relation to presenting illnesses

> *health and safety officers* and *safety representatives* to take age and disability into account in risk assessments.

STAGE 1: WHO CAN HELP AT THE 'UNSTABLE WORK' STAGE?

GP

Occupational health staff at work

Trade-union safety representatives

Work colleagues

Line managers

Family members

Citizens Advice Bureau

This first stage of work limitation is as far as it goes for workers in the growing casual sector of the labour market (e.g. migrant workers, unskilled workers in the minority ethnic communities, and workers from the newer European Union states). Agency workers or day labourers who are not able to work because of ill health are not *absent* from work, as they have no employment security. They do not as a rule qualify for Statutory Sick Pay. Migrant workers will receive only social security benefits that are immediately concerned with work. Often primary care is the first call that migrant workers make on state services. Specialist advice on social security benefits and employment rights is essential, and interpreters are also important.

THE START OF SICKNESS ABSENCE

The *first day of sickness absence* marks the start of the next stage. Most patients will self-certify their first days of time off work. Expectations of returning to work are often high, but when this will happen is not always clear. For someone who is unaccustomed to taking time off, the clinician's view is often revelatory.

At this stage there is often little contact between employer and employee. Most employers' sickness absence policies will require little more than notification by telephone if an employee is not coming in, without a procedure for contact in the short term. Phone calls will often be between the employee's partner and office staff, and are understandably brief. It is still exceptional for occupational health services to become involved at an early stage in sickness absence, and of course most patients will not have access to occupational health services at work in any case.

If there have been several recent short spells of sickness absence, a further spell will not always be dealt with sympathetically by an employer. It may raise suspicions of abuse of sick pay arrangements or even of an alcohol dependence problem. However, it may also represent a patient's way of managing a fluctuating health problem, or menstrual pain. The Bradford system of totting up periods of sickness absence to trigger investigations, however logical it may seem to managers (who find unforeseen absence difficult to cover), is often seen by patients as unfair in that it penalises multiple short periods of sickness absence by comparison with longer periods of time off taken in a single stretch.

It can be a relief to give up the struggle to remain at work. During the first weeks of sickness absence, the employee's GP, family and work colleagues (including line managers) are often the only people who know enough to help. When the employee asks for a sick note, the first formal communication between GP and workplace occurs. Even with full use of the 'comments' section on the Med 3 form, communication between the GP and the workplace at this stage is formulaic. It could be much more instrumental.

Some of the possible uses of sick notes are discussed in Chapter 4. They are reflected in patients' greater willingness to have 'work-related stress' written on a sick note (rather than 'anxiety' or 'depression' or simply 'stress'), knowing that it flags up management responsibility for conditions at work. If the diagnosis on the sick note is one of the reportable occupational diseases, the sick note should trigger investigation by the employer and possibly by the health and safety authorities. In the Sheffield practices in which occupational health advisers work, in addition to a sick note and rather than waiting for an enquiry from the employer to reach the GP practice, we ask patients whether they feel that a letter to their line manager would be useful. The letter will focus on what needs to be done at work to achieve a sustainable return to work.

The early weeks of sickness absence are a sensitive period, when non-coercive 'keeping in touch' by line managers or colleagues can prepare the way for a speedy return to work, but frequent high-pressure phone calls or text messages can have exactly the opposite effect. The worker depends heavily on contact with clinicians to grasp what might happen next, the progression of the illness and the likelihood and timing of a return to work, and hence what to tell managers and work colleagues about future developments.

This is a time when prompt medical intervention can influence the duration of sickness absence. Research has demonstrated that good clinical management of health problems leads to the most rapid return to work. Waiting for healthcare is associated with longer periods of sickness absence and movement into the third stage. GPs, trade-union representatives and other primary care workers could do more at this stage to prevent the emergence of new barriers to return to work.

The timing of progression to the third stage of sickness absence varies from one individual to another. The timing may vary, but the *second sick note* is the time to start thinking about how to prevent the third stage from occurring. It is not necessary to wait just because sickness-absence policies do not require early intervention. Research shows that during early sickness absence, a longer period off sick is predicted for patients who:

› have had long periods off sick in the recent past
› are awaiting treatment
› are older
› have lower expectations of returning to work
› have lower expectations of their work ability
› lack occupational health support at work
› are in manual jobs
› are unskilled or have lower levels of educational attainment
› are more severely affected by their main health problem

❭ have psychological health problems
❭ are from ethnic-minority groups.

The following questions need to be considered.
❭ Could changes at work make an earlier return to work possible?
❭ How could line managers, occupational health staff and other workers make this happen?
❭ Could an urgent referral for investigation or treatment be justified because of the possible consequences of a long period off work? Employers' experience suggests that it could.
❭ What should the GP say if the patient asks about seeking help privately or using complementary medicine to circumvent delays?

STAGE 2: WHO CAN HELP WHEN SICKNESS ABSENCE STARTS?

GP
Line manager
Work colleagues (by keeping in touch)
Occupational health professionals at work
Trade-union safety representatives
Occupational health advisers in primary care

CASE MANAGEMENT OR BETTER COMMUNICATION?

What happens next has been the focus of attention both in the scientific literature and in intervention studies. Most sickness absence is short term in nature. Illnesses follow their set patterns, and self-limiting conditions resolve. However, in a proportion of episodes of illness this does not happen. Longer spells of sickness absence are marked by changes in psychological attitudes on the part of the employee, and in organisational behaviour at work. The number of patients moving into long-term sickness absence may be small at any given time, but it is cumulatively large and requires disproportionate amounts of clinical and rehabilitation support.

When does this third stage start?

There is no consistency about when the third stage starts. When speaking to patients who have been off sick for a month or so, a diversity of circumstances is apparent.

Some are waiting impatiently for a fairly certain *arc of recovery* to be completed. Others are extremely uncertain about what will happen next. They could be waiting for the outcome of investigations, because the health professionals concerned have not been told that delay could be damaging. In these circumstances the patient's desire to return to work may be resolute. Attitudes at work towards the absent worker may be changing nonetheless.

Psychological changes

Other patients become depressed during periods of sickness absence, rapidly becoming so after a heart attack or other life-threatening event, and more slowly after the onset of a back problem. One interpretation of this difference is that a life-threatening condition provokes an immediate psychological response, whereas a work-limiting condition with an uncertain prognosis results in psychological changes as a result of more complex social processes at work and at home.

Financial worries

These start almost immediately for the large numbers of employees who are receiving low levels of occupational sick pay or Statutory Sick Pay only. Illness is isolating, and isolation, loss of income, fear of job loss, fatalism about the course of the illness, and loss of sustaining relationships at work all compound the physical and psychological symptoms of the illness itself. The impressive work done to change expectations of people with back pain has begun to address these changes in the Salford Back Pain Trial, and now in the Pathways to Work schemes.

The response at work

At work, the cast in this third act may include occupational health professionals, line managers, human resources personnel and trade-union representatives. At this stage employers are likely to make contact with the patient, in order to plan for sickness cover or return to work. This can be positive and helpful for employees, but it often feels threatening. Line managers may conclude that they cannot depend upon the employee's return, and the employee feels fearful about the change in attitude not only of line managers but also of work colleagues. Subtle changes of attitude reflect the fact that work colleagues and supervisors may be having to cope with an additional workload, and in the absence of better information, may question the nature of the sickness that is causing absence, particularly when it is put down to stress, depression or anxiety.

Occupational health and human resources personnel

These professionals may be following their occupational health and capability procedures. However, one thing that stands out from surveys of rehabilitation practice is that there is no consistent 'best-practice' trigger point for invoking either of these processes, which seem to the patient to be at odds with one another.

The third stage in healthcare

GPs and other clinical staff are still involved, although they may feel that the clinical recovery has been overtaken by those social and psychological processes at home and at work which they are much less confident about handling. More health professionals are likely to be playing their part, such as physiotherapists, counsellors, mental health professionals working in general practices, and others working in community or secondary care.

QUESTIONS TO ASK DURING THE THIRD STAGE

- If the patient has had (or is at risk of) a sharp drop in income, have they seen a benefits adviser?
- If the capability procedure has been started at work, is the patient being assisted by a trade-union or staff representative, and if not, have they taken a friend with them to any disciplinary hearings?
- Have occupational health professionals at work become involved, and could the Access to Work team at Jobcentre Plus help with equipment, transport to work or provision of an assistant?
- Should the patient be considering a major change of job involving retraining, vocational guidance or job hunting?

A number of people may be seeing the patient by this time, and there are some arguments in favour of a case management approach. Currently no one has a prior claim for the case management role, so as things stand no agency is resourced, or is making a strong claim, to case manage returns to work (except in those rare but severe cases of injury after a road traffic or works accident, when insurers may become involved).

Indeed it is arguable that case management should never be the method of choice. Improved communication between the workplace, clinical staff and rehabilitation professionals could obviate the need for a specific and probably costly additional case management role.

WHO CAN HELP DURING LONGER PERIODS OF SICKNESS ABSENCE?

- *Clinical staff:* GP, nurse, physiotherapist, counsellor, mental health worker.
- *Workplace:* occupational health professionals, human resources and line managers, trade-union safety representatives.
- *Community:* benefits advisers, debt counsellors, vocational guidance specialists, Access to Work team at Jobcentre Plus.

By the end of this third stage of sickness absence it makes little difference whether a patient is still employed or has become unemployed, as the probability of a return to the previous job is low. There are exceptions, and these reveal something about our attitudes to work and ill health.

Many employers will hold a job open if there is a fairly high degree of certainty about an eventual return – slow recovery from injury (especially if it occurred at work) or surgery is often accepted. Managers need certainty to plan for cover, and a relatively certain return date some months away is better than no date at all.

Using the Disability Discrimination Act

If the underlying cause of sickness absence is a disability as defined in the Disability Discrimination Act, the employer may try to make the necessary job adaptations to enable the patient to come back to work. Physical disabilities seem to be accepted more easily than mental ones. It is not overstating its importance to say that GPs' understanding of the meaning of disability in the Disability Discrimination Act will do more to help a patient with long-term health problems to remain at work than any other item of knowledge. At present only larger employers seem to be aware of the help that they can get from Access to Work teams to accommodate workers with a (Disability Discrimination Act-defined) disability.

FROM SICKNESS ABSENCE TO UNEMPLOYMENT

The final stage starts if no stable return to work has been possible. Markers for this stage include:

- the end of a 'capability' procedure (a formal investigation of long-term absence) at work involving personnel (human resources) specialists and employee representatives
- moving from Statutory Sick Pay or occupational sick pay to state benefits (normally Incapacity Benefit)

> leaving work voluntarily
> contact between the patient and Jobcentre Plus to make an Incapacity Benefit claim
> contact between Jobcentre Plus and the GP to inform the GP about the success of the Incapacity Benefit claim (and hence whether further sick notes are required).

Two new factors can now emerge, namely secondary health problems (particularly depression) and social disorientation (the sense of shock and loss of direction that comes from facing a forced change in one's working life). A few people adapt to long-term unemployment as a career change in itself, developing voluntary work or caring responsibilities to acquire a new sense of purpose, but for those who are most vulnerable – that is, former manual workers without transferable skills to get around their limiting health problem – the choices are stark and limited. It would be desirable for training options to be available to help them, but the cost of training, as well as the risk of losing state benefits by starting to retrain, means that this is rarely a viable course of action.

Changing jobs

There is very little difference between the situation of an employee who has been off sick for a long time and faces redeployment, dismissal or leaving voluntarily, and the situation of someone who is already out of work. The benefits situation is almost the same – they are likely to be on Incapacity Benefit and means-tested benefits if they are eligible. To have remained off sick for long enough (normally 28 weeks) to qualify for Incapacity Benefit, they are unlikely to be able to return to the kind of work they were previously doing. Their needs for advice and support are very similar. In addition to continuing clinical management by GPs and other health professionals, people who have been out of work for as long as this may need support into alternative work.

Support needs

The support that is required at this stage is quite different to that described above. Help with financial problems, vocational guidance, support with job finding, specialist assessment and training all play a part. It is exceptional for these to be provided primarily by an employer. The largest corporate employers have a sufficient range of jobs and turnover to redeploy staff, but even in this case redeployment is poorly coordinated. Line management, occupational health staff, human resources departments and trade-union representatives often seem to have their own goals and do not always work well together, and the organisation of labour into competing pools in large companies may prevent this in any case.

As a result, in this final stage, the range of potential helpers has expanded again. The voluntary sector's many providers of job-finding and in-work support could become involved, along with the Department for Work and Pensions Disability Employment Advisers (DEAs). Good advice on benefits is essential. In our work in primary care, advisers from Sheffield Occupational Health Advisory Service have found that many adults need vocational guidance, as a change of job is often the only way out of their predicament. The relevant agencies include vocational guidance specialists ('careers advisers'), job-finding agencies, including Jobcentre Plus, and the voluntary-sector support agencies and DEAs mentioned above.

Patients who move on to Incapacity Benefit or who are assessed as being entitled to the new Rehabilitation Support Allowance may be able to access an integrated service of the kind piloted by Pathways to Work schemes. The route to this kind of help is currently via the patient's personal adviser at Jobcentre Plus.

WHO CAN HELP WHEN SICKNESS ABSENCE BECOMES UNEMPLOYMENT?

Clinical staff: GP, nurse, physiotherapist, counsellor.
Workplace: human resources managers, occupational health professionals, trade-union representatives, line managers.
Community: benefits advisers, debt counsellors, vocational guidance specialists, employment law specialists, Disability Employment Advisers at Jobcentre Plus, Job Support projects, specialist voluntary-sector job support, voluntary work agencies, local training providers.

WHO'S WHO IN JOB RETENTION AND RETURN TO WORK

The cast is large (*see* Table 5.1). There are three main spheres of activity, namely the workplace, the health services and the job support sector. Working on the government's Job Retention and Rehabilitation Pilot drew my attention to the way in which each group has its own purposes, procedures and endpoints. Larger workplaces have employment practices laid down as a series of policies linked to the employment contract. Procedures have to be followed with the aim of getting the individual to become a productive employee again.

Table 5.1 Where to find help

WORKPLACE	TIPS FOR UTILISATION
Human resource (HR) departments	Smaller firms don't have them, large firms have HR departments at headquarters – not always accessible from branches, subsidiary companies, etc.
Health and safety managers	As above
Occupational health departments	Increasingly contracted out; the patient may not know how to contact them directly
Line managers	Ask the patient for the name and department, and address letters to them directly
Trade-union representatives (shop stewards or safety representatives)	Suggest that the patient involves the trade-union representative, or failing that a full-time official of the union
COMMUNITY	
Benefits advisers and debt counsellors	Citizens Advice Bureaux, specialist advisers (mental health, Age Concern, migrant workers and refugees), some outreach in primary care premises
Vocational guidance specialists	Career services or new providers; no systematic way of finding them
Disability Employment Advisers	Jobcentre Plus
Access to Work teams	Jobcentre Plus regional call centre
Job Support projects	Various private- or voluntary-sector job-finding agencies (including Remploy, Employment Opportunities for People with Disabilities, Shaw Trust); Department for Work and Pensions website
Specialist voluntary sector job support (RNID, RNIB, learning difficulties, mental health)	Department for Work and Pensions website; national websites of charities
Voluntary work agencies	Local councils for voluntary service or similar
Universities, further education colleges	All have disability specialists (see websites)
HEALTH	
Occupational therapists	Community mental health teams, hospital hand clinics, cardiovascular rehabilitation teams, etc.
Social workers	Community mental health teams
Social inclusion workers	Mental health day services
Employment advisers, occupational health advisers	A few pilot projects and small-scale services

Health services are little better than the workplace, for they are driven by the need to reach a point at which a patient can either be discharged, or ceases to consult. Return to work has not been routinely taken into account by health professionals, and barely figures in the NHS targets and service frameworks. GPs and hospital specialists will inevitably have given opinions about when a patient should be fit to return to work, but the NHS has not prioritised making sure that the relevant treatments and investigations are available when they are needed, so as not to put the patient's job at risk. The need for health professionals to have a deeper knowledge of what a particular job involves and of the complex relationships between occupation and health is only now being recognised.

The job-finding and job-support sector engages with people who are off sick or unemployed as clients whose progress and eventual stable return to work may help them to achieve the targets upon which their contracts depend.

WORKING TOGETHER

If different professional contributions are to support one another, they require mutual understanding. Dutch academics have tried to improve the relationships between work-based occupational physicians and family doctors, recognising that if each holds the other in low regard there is a risk that their approaches to sickness absence will conflict with each other. And that is just one relationship. What can be done to give everyone involved a common sense of purpose?

One step forward . . .

Political leadership helps. My impression is that the government's focus on sickness absence over the past few years *has* brought about changes of attitude, but not always in the same direction. Line managers are often under such pressure to deliver set targets that the best intentions of occupational health specialists and GPs in asking for modified work responsibilities are soon frustrated. Capability procedures and good occupational health practice have different timescales and are often at odds with one another, and I have gained the impression that in many medium-sized enterprises redeployment is nobody's responsibility.

More providers

The diversity of skills required to help patients who wish to return to work determines the overall approach that is taken in primary care. Primary care has good access to clinical skills, but depends for other rehabilitation support on private- and public-sector services. However, the information that is required in order to refer appropriately in the full knowledge of referral criteria, waiting times, skills and intended outcomes is beyond the means of most health professionals and workplace occupational health and human resource departments.

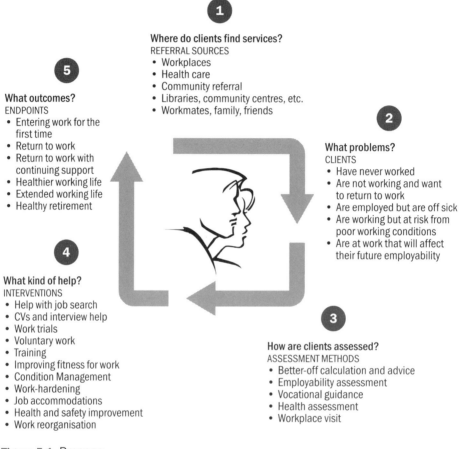

1

Where do clients find services?
REFERRAL SOURCES
• Workplaces
• Health care
• Community referral
• Libraries, community centres, etc.
• Workmates, family, friends

5

What outcomes?
ENDPOINTS
• Entering work for the first time
• Return to work
• Return to work with continuing support
• Healthier working life
• Extended working life
• Healthy retirement

2

What problems?
CLIENTS
• Have never worked
• Are not working and want to return to work
• Are employed but are off sick
• Are working but at risk from poor working conditions
• Are at work that will affect their future employability

4

What kind of help?
INTERVENTIONS
• Help with job search
• CVs and interview help
• Work trials
• Voluntary work
• Training
• Improving fitness for work
• Condition Management
• Work-hardening
• Job accommodations
• Health and safety improvement
• Work reorganisation

3

How are clients assessed?
ASSESSMENT METHODS
• Better-off calculation and advice
• Employability assessment
• Vocational guidance
• Health assessment
• Workplace visit

Figure 5.1 Process.

The range of providers in the job-support and job-finding sector is continuing to expand. The success of the Salford Back Pain Project and the popularity of Condition Management Programmes as part of the government's Pathways to Work programme highlight the importance of support that harnesses several different kinds of professional skills. These include vocational guidance, training advice, job-finding services, in-work support, physical therapies (including physiotherapy and occupational therapy) and psychological therapies. Together they make up a constellation of services, with stars of different and varying magnitudes, and it is hard for anyone – in the health service or the workplace – to see what is available at a particular time. Mapping the services becomes a time-consuming service in itself, particularly when providers are on short-term contracts. There is a serious problem with regard to coordination and fitness for purpose here.

It may take years to develop an integrated approach to rehabilitation among the many providers of support (*see* Figure 5.1).

One approach to resolving the issue of multiple interventions and agencies has been to develop an occupational health or employment and health role in primary care, if not to provide a case management service, then at least to advise patients and clinicians about what is available.

USE OF MULTIPLE INTERVENTIONS AND AGENCIES

This requires:

- a clear understanding of what services are available
- up-to-date information on referral criteria, waiting times and contact details
- effective two-way communication to ensure that patients reach the service and are receiving the help planned
- mutual respect among professionals, with recognition of individual strengths and weaknesses, complementarity and duplication
- a coordination or case management role for people with complex needs
- a stepped approach to ensure that only those who need high-input interventions are receiving them
- clarity about who is doing what and when, including who is responsible for the coordination role.

A NEW ROLE IN PRIMARY CARE

Over the last 25 years a number of primary care-based services have developed to deal with work/health issues. The role that the services take on has broadened from a traditional occupational disease prevention model (offering advice to people with health problems caused by work) to a comprehensive model that covers the various interfaces between employment and health.

The most common approach is for the adviser to take referrals from clinical staff and others at clinic sessions in GP surgeries several times each month. The occupational health adviser is able to provide a stepped or 'tiered' intervention appropriate to each case. This could range from advice or referral, or more time-consuming interventions such as health surveillance or drafting letters to employers, through to full-blown case management with workplace visits and support after the return to work.

Evaluations of the non-medical primary care adviser services show that they lead to successful return to work, improved working conditions and reductions in GP consultations. However, the occupational health advisory service has been difficult to replicate outside a few pioneer centres (Sheffield, Rotherham, Leeds, Liverpool and formerly others). No single source of funding from within the NHS has been identified to provide this service on a long-term basis. A more recent innovation has been the employment adviser initiative funded by the Department for Work and Pensions (*see* Chapter 4). GPs have been enthusiastic about the potential of Pathways to Work and similar schemes to help their patients, and are happy to refer patients to an employment adviser who is working on their premises.

The underlying insights here are that primary care is accessible to patients, well trusted and an early point of contact for people with work-limiting illnesses. Communication between work and primary care has in the past been minimal (sick notes, or letters from human resources or occupational health departments at a late stage), and can easily be improved upon.

In the Sheffield service, we aim to communicate early, clarifying what might be needed to enable a patient to return to work quickly. The best time for this is probably around the time of the second sick note, before problems become chronic. A letter is often sufficient, but we also find that employers are happy for us to visit the workplace and to have a three-way discussion with the employee/patient present when the issues are more complicated.

PATIENTS WITH MENTAL HEALTH PROBLEMS OR WORK-RELATED STRESS NEED SPECIAL HELP

There are two reasons for giving separate consideration to the return-to-work support needed by people suffering from work-related stress or mental health problems. The first is that they both affect the very relationships at work which permit and sustain return-to-work interventions. The second reason is that– perhaps because of this – we know little about the kind of help that is most likely to be successful.

In another sense all long-term sickness absence is concerned with mental health problems. Analysis of sickness absence in the past considered the decision to take time off from work as a psychological process of withdrawal from the workplace. This interpretation has been largely forgotten, as sickness absence has come to be viewed more as a form of transgression against the norm of participating in society through work. Time off from work is also a time of additional anxieties – about money, working relationships, family relationships, loss of social standing, and the uncertainty of the sick role.

Stress

Even the word 'stress' upsets some occupational health professionals. It seems ill defined or ambiguous. This is, I believe, its attraction. It is a lay term which captures the way that relationships at work, and the demands of work, affect us psychologically and physiologically or 'biopsychosocially.' At work, in addition to meeting their material needs, people try to meet various psychological needs – for social recognition, the satisfaction of achievement, self-realisation, social engagement, and an expectation that the organisation will honour its duty of care.

When patients report that they are suffering from stress, the relationships that need to be in place to make a return to work a success, namely support from a line manager and colleagues, and positive and consistent commitment from the patient, are in doubt. So what works?

What works?

The government's flagship Job Retention and Rehabilitation Pilot found that patients with mental health problems were the most difficult to assist with returning to work. The findings had more serious implications. Trying to help in these circumstances even seems to have had the effect of hindering. Patients who received no help (the control group in the research) were more likely to have returned to work than those who received interventions, but to have done so by changing their job. My interpretation of these findings is that when workplace relationships have broken down – and it is worth remembering that half of the Job Retention and Rehabilitation Pilot clients first received help 12 weeks after the first day of sickness absence – it is best to look for work elsewhere. As an occupational health manager said to me, 'We think Joe should return to work – but not here.'

This implies, of course, that the range of services that clients need is more akin to that required by those who have been absent from work for long periods, namely job-finding help, vocational guidance help with benefits, etc. In addition, because a breakdown of relationships will often be perceived by the employee as being due to unreasonable behaviour on the part of a manager or work colleague, dispute resolution skills may also be needed (although these have yet to be formally evaluated).

Some obstacles

A sense of injustice may delay the inevitable. In this situation, justice in its purest, compensatory and retributive form is hard to obtain. Constructive dismissal (where an employer is held to have behaved in a way that left the employee with no alternative but to leave the job) is difficult to prove and will normally only be held to have occurred where an employee has first gone through the employer's grievance procedure. Delays are almost inevitable. Patients and their advisers – who should be union representatives, or legal or paralegal employment rights advisers – should help the patient to weigh up the options. A sense of injustice but a quick release is often to be preferred to a sense of partial justice and a protracted conflict, which is stressful in itself.

Patients' own patterns of behaviour can contribute to stress – for example, by lacking assertiveness or being too combative, by over- or under-commitment to work, by pre-occupation with matters in the family or home environment, etc. Dealing with problems of this kind or with common mental health problems such as depression or anxiety means integrating appropriate therapies into the return-to-work process. These are often in short supply. Larger employers may provide some counselling or even cognitive–behavioural therapy, or better-off patients may be able to pay for treatment, but for most patients the limited availability of such therapies – and the length of time that they take to become effective – may put a job at risk.

However, it is worth remembering that chronic mental health problems are likely to be considered a disability under the Disability Discrimination Act. This means that even if an employee has been off sick for months, their employer must take a reasonable approach to accommodating the employee's disability-related needs. The capability procedure must take disability into account.

OVERCOMING THE OBSTACLES

Severe mental health problems are a common cause of unemployment. The problems described earlier in relation to common mental health problems are compounded. A patient who is out of work and has moderate to severe mental health problems is at a disadvantage when trying to start work for many reasons.

Changing attitudes and expectations

In terms of attitudes and temperament the patient may be far from what employers are looking for. He or she may have little confidence, motivation or work ethic, and may well lack the stamina and concentration required for full-time work. Expectation of unfavourable treatment, whether based on experience or not, can lead people to use strategies for finding work that are unlikely to succeed. Everyone involved in the patient's rehabilitation needs to help to increase that person's confidence, motivation and stamina, and to bear in mind that lack of a work ethic may be the consequence of a long period of inactivity.

Acquiring the skills necessary to find and stay in work

In addition to the obvious skills that come from a consistent history of education, training and previous work, there are core skills of social engagement, assertiveness and autonomy that are assumed in many jobs. Life skills such as being sufficiently organised to get ready to work each day may have been lost during a period of debilitating mental illness.

Managing mood

Although consistency of mood is an unrealistic expectation of any employee, there is no doubt that protracted periods of anxiety or low mood make demands on fellow workers and may make an individual less attractive as a (potential) employee. Any service provision or productive process requires a degree of stability in the behaviour of employees, and unpredictable fluctuations of mood can be detrimental. Help is needed to address anxiety and stress directly, but also to challenge the underlying causes, which may include lack of support from co-workers, or from close relationships outside work, as well as poor physical health.

Acquiring the basics for job finding

Employers make an assessment of a job applicant based on their CV, references, interview performance and possibly some task-based assessment. Anyone who has been out of work for a long period is likely to have poor interview skills, to have gaps in their CV (if they have one), and to find it difficult to obtain suitable references. Unrealistic expectations at interview are also a problem. Past experiences of work may have been negative, but the patient will nevertheless feel that they should be treated fairly. Patients sometimes expect to be able to manage a demanding full-time post in the hope of solving financial problems, when a gradual return to work would be more likely to succeed. Vocational guidance for adults is in short supply, but local careers services and job-finding agencies may provide some help.

Help with financial problems

Any long period of unemployment will be marked by relatively low income. Difficulties in managing the balancing act to remain solvent (whether on a low income or not) may have resulted in serious debt problems. Some people take on unrealistic amounts of work in the hope of overcoming their debt burden, while others may move house frequently or even become homeless, which means that the secure base required for a demanding full-time job is often not there.

Developing working relationships

The process of returning to work requires gradual establishment of patterns of occupation – often voluntary work or work placements – en route to a conventional job. Potential employers need to be prepared prior to interview to deal fairly with an applicant who has a fractured employment history and fragile self-confidence. The workforce needs to have mental health awareness training in order to avoid attitudes that put a new appointee at an immediate disadvantage.

WHO CAN HELP PATIENTS WITH MENTAL HEALTH PROBLEMS TO RETURN TO WORK?

- Voluntary work and training providers can help patients to develop vocational skills.
- Educational establishments have specific disability support that can be crucial while skills and qualifications are being acquired.
- Adult guidance and job-finding agencies can help with CV writing and honing the skills needed during appointment processes.
- Specialist agencies such as the Disability Employment Advisers (DEAs) at Jobcentre Plus or the Sheffield User Employment Project (which helps mental health service users to re-enter employment) can help to establish working relationships by preparing potential employers for non-discriminatory recruitment, and organising work placements and work trials.
- Clinicians contribute by adopting best clinical practice for managing mental health problems and establishing the solid basis of stable moods and predictable behaviour necessary for work.
- Mental health staff (e.g. social workers, social inclusion workers, day centre staff, occupational therapists) can help with signposting and case managing.
- Trainers can help workforces to be more aware of the needs of employees with chronic mental health problems.

- Health and safety officials and human resources departments need to address unhealthy working relationships within the government's Stress Management Standards format.
- Benefits advisers, debt support workers and DEAs will need to provide advice on managing finances during a work trial. Alternatively, going on a work placement could form part of the strategy of maximising income during a gradual return to full-time work.

WHAT ARE THE OUTCOMES?

With so many different needs, it is not surprising that starting work is often a long process for people with mental health problems, and that staying in work requires more support than might be needed for individuals whose work-limiting health problems are mainly physical. Success rates are likely to be quite low (one charity has reported that only 10% of its caseload move into work each year), but small steps that reduce social isolation, such as voluntary work and training, are of value both in themselves and for their contribution to the patient's health. Return to work isn't everything!

FURTHER READING

Tuomi K, Ilmarinen J, Jahkola A *et al. Work Ability Index.* Helsinki: Finnish Institute of Occupational Health; 1998.

CHAPTER 6

Assessment of fitness for work in practice

FITNESS FOR WORK: GENERAL PRINCIPLES

The clinical assessment of fitness for work aims to ensure that individuals are physically and mentally able to do all the tasks expected of them, without risk to themselves or to others.

An individual's health status may affect their physical or emotional capacity for work, and the job itself may be known to cause health problems or to exacerbate existing ones. In either situation, it may not be medically appropriate for someone to attempt a particular job. For some jobs there may be specific advisory or statutory 'fitness standards.'

➤ Medical conditions may make an employee physically incapable of performing a job efficiently for the employer and safely for the employee. For example:
  - a person with chronic musculoskeletal problems may be unfit to do heavy manual work because of reduced mobility or strength
  - a person with ischaemic heart disease may be physically incapable of undertaking strenuous work, or working in hot conditions, without developing angina.

➤ Certain jobs may exacerbate an underlying condition. For example:
  - a person with asthma may be unfit to work in dust or fumes
  - a person with insulin-dependent diabetes may be unfit to work in a strenuous job where meal breaks and rest breaks are unpredictable.

➤ Medical conditions can affect the health and safety of others. For example:

- a person with epilepsy may be unfit to drive or to climb
- a person with chronic skin disease may be unfit to work in a job that involves food preparation
- a person with poorly controlled psychiatric problems may not be fit to drive a train, because of the potential for abnormal behaviour.

PRACTICAL ASSESSMENT OF FITNESS FOR WORK

To make an informed assessment of fitness for work, particularly in the case of an individual who is out of work or changing their job, we need to know enough about:

) the individual's medical conditions
) how those conditions affect their functional capacity
) what the current (and proposed) medical treatments are
) how medical treatment might affect the individual's capacity for work
) the physical and emotional requirements of the job, in order to anticipate (as objectively as possible) how the individual's capacity or health may be affected at work.

Assessment should always be related to the job in question. There is really no such thing as 'general' fitness for work. Most people are capable of doing something productive, even though their limitations may be quite severe (ask Professor Stephen Hawking!).

The GP, practice nurse or hospital doctor usually knows enough about an individual's medical conditions and their treatment, but it is often knowledge of the requirements of particular jobs that is lacking. This can lead to the issuing of inappropriate advice on fitness for work, either because certain demands or risks inherent in the job are not understood, or because the doctor or nurse chooses to be overcautious, advising a patient not to attempt a job, with little supporting evidence.

WHAT IS AN 'OCCUPATION'?

To decide whether someone is medically fit – that is, to assess *functional capacity* in real detail – we might want to divide an 'occupation' into the following elements:

) *job* – a group of 'duties' performed by one person, often as part of a team
) *task* – a discrete unit of work performed by one individual, usually consisting of a logical and necessary step in the performance of a duty,

with an identifiable beginning and end
) *task element* – the smallest step into which it is possible to subdivide any
   work activity, without analysing separate movements.

This kind of detailed analysis is not usually necessary in practice, even for
occupational health professionals, but where someone has a particular medical
problem (e.g. a musculoskeletal problem) it may be necessary to think about
which tasks or even task elements might cause problems.

MEDICAL STANDARDS OF FITNESS

Specific medical standards apply to certain jobs, and may be advisory or
statutory.
) Well-known *statutory* fitness standards include those for professional
   drivers (Large Goods Vehicles and Passenger-Carrying Vehicles), and for
   pilots and seafarers.
) *Advisory* standards apply in certain industries, and may be developed
   largely by the industry itself (e.g. food handling and production) or may
   be developed by other agencies, such as the Health and Safety Executive
   (e.g. driving forklift trucks).

Many of these medical standards have been developed in a 'health and
safety' context, largely in order to protect other people (e.g. work colleagues,
customers, the public). Medical standards for professional drivers take into
account the risk of a medical condition causing sudden incapacity and risk to
other road users. Similar assessments apply to pilots and train drivers. Fitness
standards for food handlers are aimed at protecting consumers, and standards
for healthcare workers are at least partly aimed at protecting patients.
   Where there is no statutory standard, occupational health physicians may
apply relevant standards derived by analogy from published or statutory
standards. For example, school crossing patrols might be expected to have
equivalent eyesight to the drivers whom they are directing. However, when
applying standards, practitioners need to be reasonable and to avoid the
challenge that they might be discriminatory with regard to age, gender or
disability.

ASSESSMENT FRAMEWORK

As in any medical assessment, a systematic approach is helpful, taking into account the following:

> stamina and liability to fatigue
> mobility, range of movements of joints and spine, and difficulties with certain postures (e.g. sitting, stooping, bending)
> strength, dexterity, coordination and balance
> cardiorespiratory problems and exercise tolerance – tendency to exacerbations of angina, breathlessness
> neurological problems – liability to sudden unconsciousness or incapacity
> sensory and communication problems – vision, hearing, speech
> neuropsychological and psychiatric problems – memory, intellect, behaviour and motivation
> medical treatments, including possible side-effects (drowsiness, fluid/electrolyte disturbances)
> special needs (e.g. diabetes, stomas) that might require organisational adjustments – meal breaks, access to medication, access to toilet facilities, particular aids in the workplace.

This list is not exhaustive, but neither will all of these potential problems relate to every job. A sedentary office job in a clean environment is obviously very different to a job as a firefighter.

Some basic examples will now be considered.

The forklift truck driver

Pete Jones is 56 years old, and has applied for a job as a forklift truck (FLT) driver in a warehouse, after a period of unemployment. He is keen to return to work. He has a history of type 2 diabetes mellitus, controlled with oral hypoglycaemic medication, longstanding back and neck pain and some osteoarthritis in his hands, but only takes a few paracetamol for this. He has not needed non-steroidal anti-inflammatory drugs (NSAIDs) for 2 years – the last time his low back pain flared up. He has no other medical conditions that we are aware of (in particular, no cardiovascular disease and no neurological problems).

What else do we need to know to help to determine his fitness for this job? Are there any guidelines on fitness to drive a FLT?

The Health and Safety Executive publishes guidelines on medical fitness [HS(G)6], and although these are not a legal requirement, like all such guidance, the Courts would expect these standards to be applied, or at least something demonstrably equivalent to them.

How might Pete's medical conditions affect his physical capacity? His diabetes might cause problems in the workplace, but only if he is prone to hyper- or hypoglycaemia. As far as we know, his diabetic control is good on oral medication and diet. Is his vision still good? Is his hearing adequate to hear other vehicles and warnings?

His musculoskeletal problems may be more significant. Is he fully mobile? Can he walk easily – or even run short distances in an emergency? Are his grip strength and reach reasonable, and does this matter? Is his back pain well controlled, so that he can sit on a truck for prolonged periods? Are his neck movements normal?

Driving an FLT generates certain musculoskeletal stresses and strains. He will need to be able to turn his head and to look up without difficulty. FLT drivers often drive backwards, looking over their shoulders, and may need to manipulate very heavy objects on their forks, either from or to a high rack. A person who can't look up easily, or move their head quickly, might endanger himself and others.

Can he grip, lift and pull? Obviously he will need to be able to work the controls of his truck, but is he just going to be driving? Warehouse operatives often have to 'pick' items by hand as well as drive trucks, so can he lift boxes from low-level racks, or from above his head, safely and repeatedly?

What about his back pain? Warehouses often have uneven floors, and however well sprung the seat of his truck may be, he will be exposed to whole-body vibration as he drives. This may aggravate low back pain, as may awkward twisting postures.

However, let's not be too pessimistic, bearing in mind that Pete appears to be well motivated, and if we tell him that his back and neck ache make him unfit for the job, we may be relegating him to a prolonged and fruitless job search. He is only 'unfit' if we really think there are safety implications arising from his musculoskeletal conditions.

In general, detailed advice on fitness to drive an FLT is derived from the standards for ordinary driving licence holders in *Medical Aspects of Fitness to Drive* (published by the Department for Transport), with some fairly obvious areas of concern.

The baker

Janet Collins is 33 years old, and wants to go to work in a high-street bakery shop. She had ulcerative colitis for many years, and has been unable to work for the last 2 years, initially because of the colitis, and then because she had an ileostomy.

Is she fit to work with food? What problems might be associated with work in a high-street food shop?
If she has learned to cope with her ileostomy, and it is well controlled (i.e. not prone to leakage, etc.), there is no reason why she shouldn't work in the shop from a food hygiene point of view. Obviously she will need access to toilet facilities (and privacy), but the bacterial content of ileostomy fluid is significantly lower than that of normal faeces, so with good personal hygiene Janet will not be a 'risk' to her customers.

Are there any other factors that we need to take into account?
High-street bakeries may be hot places to work – often baking whole trays of pies and pastries. Janet may be at a small risk of dehydration from her ileostomy and the hot conditions, so will need to keep up her fluid intake. She may also have to handle heavy trays, sometimes close to her body, so she will need to take care with her stoma. However, these issues should not be insuperable.

Fitness to work as a food handler is the subject of some general advice,[1] and there may also be industry-specific guidance. The main problems arise with skin disease (chronic eczema of the hands, chronic otitis externa, flaking psoriasis). These conditions tend to be colonised with *Staphyloccocus aureus* and other organisms, with the risk of transmission of food poisoning, particularly through uncooked foods (cream products, etc.). Carriers of *Salmonella* species (particularly *S. typhi*) need to be excluded from food handling until excretion has been eliminated. However, in general it is not necessary to stool test a potential employee before work in the food industry (or after an acute gastro-intestinal illness) unless there is a real suspicion of infection with *Salmonella*, *Campylobacter* or other serious food-poisoning organisms.

The firefighter

Bill Harrison is 51 years old, and has been a firefighter for 22 years. Before that he was a painter and decorator. Over the past 5 years he has had increasing problems with his right knee. He had cartilage removed (due to a football injury) in his early thirties, and more recently he has had stiffness, pain and swelling in the knee. He has asked his orthopaedic surgeon for a knee joint replacement.

Can he go on working as a firefighter? Would he be able to go back to operational duties even if he could persuade his surgeon to do a joint replacement at his age?

The real problems here relate to fitness to work in a very physically demanding environment. Climbing, crawling, lifting and carrying all place stresses on the knee joint. It is likely that Bill's job is actually going to make his knee problems worse, by accelerating the degenerative process. Even if he has coped so far, the unpredictable nature of the job, and his colleagues' dependence on his mobility, mean that he may place others at risk, as well as himself.

It is also unlikely that a surgeon would perform a knee joint replacement at his age, but even if they did, he would be advised not to go back to heavy manual work.

This looks like a case for permanent withdrawal from operational duties, or ill health retirement from the Fire Service.

Assessing medical fitness to work in the Fire Service is often complex, requiring specific fitness testing, and is usually left to Brigade medical advisers, supported by guidance from professional organisations such as the Association of Local Authority Medical Advisers (ALAMA), and the Office of the Deputy Prime Minister. Rehabilitating a firefighter after illness or injury often requires a multi-disciplinary approach, taking into account all of the potential problems of routine and emergency work. We could easily predict what kinds of conditions might cause problems – including any difficulty with mobility, any sudden loss of consciousness or other neurological problems, cardiorespiratory problems, etc. And we should not forget the potential effects of medication. An individual

who is on a diuretic, working in hot conditions, may be more prone
to fluid and electrolyte disturbance.

THE YOUNG WORKER

Young people who are over school-leaving age and under 18 years are known
as *young workers*. At present, young people can leave school on the last Friday
of June of the school year in which they are 16 years old, although there are
indications that the school-leaving age may be raised to 18 years.

There are special laws to protect the employment rights of young workers.
These concern health and safety, what jobs they can do, when they can work,
and how many hours they can work. For example, people under school-
leaving age are not permitted to work in a factory, in construction work or in
a mine. The law recognises that young workers may be at particular risk at
work because of their possible physical and psychological immaturity and lack
of awareness of work risks, and lack of training.

An employer *must* undertake an assessment of possible risks to the health
and safety of a young worker. They must pay particular attention to *age, lack
of experience* and *specific hazards*. For young people under school-leaving age,
the employer must also tell one of the parents the results of the assessment,
including any risks identified, and any measures put in place to protect health
and safety at work. Health and safety assessments are not required for short-
term or occasional work in a family business or in a private household, if it is
not considered to be harmful.

Medical advice to young people leaving education and taking up employment
needs to be accurate, consistent and evidence based.

Consider the following example:

> Gillian is 16 years old and asks you about a career in nursing. She
> has severe atopic eczema, particularly affecting her hands, and you
> have been treating her for years with a variety of topical prepara-
> tions, without ever really getting rid of the eczema.
>
> The truth is that Gillian would have problems in nursing. Repeated
> hand-washing, use of gloves, exposure to chemicals, etc., is likely to
> exacerbate her eczema. Furthermore, if she has cracking eczema,
> she is at increased risk of acquiring infections (particularly blood-
> borne viruses), and her skin may become secondarily infected with
> *Staphylococcus aureus*, including MRSA.
>
> She should be counselled against a career in nursing. Certain

other careers, such as hairdressing (with exposures to wet chemicals, gloves, etc.) and food processing or bar work may also be
inadvisable.

In addition, prejudice needs to be tackled. This may range from an employer
believing that a diabetic will always be off work, through to a belief that
a medical student who is HIV positive should not qualify or practise as a
doctor.

Disability discrimination legislation is most helpful in assisting with a rational
and evidence-based approach to careers advice and 'fitness for work.'

In terms of risks that are specific to younger workers, there is some evidence
that musculoskeletal problems are more common. It is unclear whether this
is because younger workers tend to be given jobs that are more physically
demanding, or that are ergonomically badly designed, or because young
people are more intrinsically at risk. Accident rates in younger workers
tend to be higher, again probably linked to lack of experience, training or
supervision.

THE OLDER WORKER

In the UK, until recently the retirement age has conventionally been thought
of as 65 years for men and 60 years for women (the ages at which state
pension benefits can be drawn). However, the trend towards earlier retirement
from full-time work has been growing, with many workers opting to at least
reduce their work (if not cease economic activity altogether) before the age of
60 years. Whether there will be a sustained reversal of this trend, with financial
pressures, longer (and bigger) mortgages or loans, and changes in pension
schemes, remains to be seen.

Against this, we now have an ageing population. The post-World War Two
'Baby Boomer' generation is now the ageing workforce of the industrialised
world, generating significant financial pressures on social security and pensions
systems, and political exhortations to consider working longer – perhaps to
67 years or beyond. This advice is based largely on financial rather than cultural
pressures, using the argument of increased life expectancy as a justification.
Age discrimination legislation already enshrines the right of an employee to
work to the age of 65 years if they choose, subject only to risk-based (not age-
related) medical assessment.

What are the implications of medical fitness in relation to the older worker?
Indeed, how old is an older worker? Are they 35, 45 or 65 years of age?

General considerations

The use of spectacles, and particularly reading glasses, bifocals and varifocals increases after the age of 45 years or so, and is almost universal by the age of 55 years. This may require particular adaptations to the workplace, whether these are in computer workstation design (to take account of focusing distance) or in the ergonomics of other tasks requiring fine manual dexterity and good eyesight, such as electronic assembly work.

Age-associated hearing loss may necessitate aids to hearing that are designed with the individual's specific job in mind. For example, in-ear digital aids may be necessary for workers who need to wear helmets or other head protection. Assessment of visual acuity and hearing in relation to specific jobs therefore becomes more important as the worker ages.

Physical considerations

Age-associated changes in the body occur progressively from the age of 20 years, including changes in strength, stamina, pulmonary and cardiac function and psychomotor performance. Musculoskeletal problems increase more rapidly over the age of 45 years. However, the variation between individuals also widens, with general physical fitness, exercise, smoking and (probably) diet contributing to the overall maintenance of function. Physical strength and aerobic capacity are greatest somewhere between 20 and 30 years of age, and are subsequently lost at the rate of about 1.5% per year. The losses in strength tend to be larger in the lower than in the upper limbs. Although physical conditioning can improve baseline levels, this gradual loss occurs in Olympic athletes as well as in 'normal' workers.

It therefore follows that heavy manual work is less likely to be tolerated by older workers because of reduced stamina and strength, together with increased degenerative disease (arthritis, etc.). Some older workers may cope with heavy manual work well into their sixties, but this is unusual. Physical exercise and training have a positive effect on physical capacity ('use it or lose it'), but work in itself may not be enough to maintain fitness levels.

As physical capacity decreases, the risk of injury from accidents or overuse increases.

Memory and psychomotor performance decline with age, and this occurs more quickly in some people than in others. Reduced reaction times and slower cognitive functioning may lead to increased risks in workplaces where quickly moving machinery or other changing hazards are present. On the other hand, greater experience often offsets slower cognitive functioning, leading to similar or even better performance and lower accident rates among older workers in some jobs.

In addition to these general issues, some specific problems arise in all older workers, including changes in vision and hearing that may require adaptations at work.

The ability of someone to continue working productively and safely as they age (particularly beyond the age of 50 years) is therefore dependent on a complex set of physical, mental, environmental and cultural determinants. At its simplest, heavy manual work becomes less tolerable, jobs that are emotionally and cognitively demanding may become less easy to perform efficiently and successfully, and the ability to cope with adverse working environments (shift work, heat, cold, confined spaces, awkward postures, etc.) decreases.

Very rapidly paced work combined with mentally difficult tasks will – in theory – become difficult or impossible for older workers, but as most work does not require maximum physical or mental capacity, an older worker may simply need to work closer to maximum than a younger one. That worker may still be quite capable of fulfilling all of their job responsibilities, so long as the targets are 'reasonable.' Alongside individual problems, society and cultural pressures still encourage people to think of 'early retirement' as a good thing, perhaps encouraging the view that work is inherently bad, rather than inherently positive and beneficial for the older person.

Employers will have to take these problems into account when planning for the older worker, and this will require cultural and organisational changes that are largely beyond the control of the medical professions. There will need to be changes to shift patterns, changes to physical and ergonomic demands, job rotation, mechanisation, retraining and flexible working practices.

However, we can help by looking positively at the older worker in terms of functional capacity, advising on physical limitations where appropriate, and identifying cognitive or psychological problems, but also encouraging the older worker to believe that productive ageing is normal.

THE PREGNANT WORKER

Pregnant workers are specifically covered in UK employment and health and safety legislation. In essence, it is unlawful to discriminate against a woman in any way because of her pregnancy, and specific risk assessments need to be undertaken in relation to work.

Having said that, pregnancy should not in itself be regarded a disease or disability, or as a cause of incapacity for work. A woman may be incapable of doing a particular job if doing so would put her or her unborn child at risk, or if she suffers from complications of pregnancy (e.g. hyperemesis, hypertension, diabetes, exacerbation of musculoskeletal problems, etc.).

There are some workplace hazards that need to be considered specifically in relation to pregnancy.

Physical hazards
- *Shift work* may cause excessive tiredness in the later stages of pregnancy, and there is some evidence of increased risk of miscarriage, premature labour and low birth weight in shift workers.
- *Moving and handling* may become difficult in pregnancy, and may be associated with pre-term delivery.
- *Ionising radiation* must be avoided.
- *Hot conditions* may be more fatiguing in pregnancy.

Chemical hazards
- *Lead* is teratogenic (as well as being associated with miscarriage and stillbirth), and work with lead must be avoided in pregnancy.
- *Other chemicals* may be teratogenic or harmful to breastfed infants.
- *Risk assessment* in accordance with the principles of the Control of Substances Hazardous to Health (COSHH) Regulations must be undertaken for pregnant and breastfeeding mothers. A formal COSHH assessment must be undertaken wherever these chemicals are used, and its findings must be made available to the employee.

Biological hazards
- Specific biological hazards that must be avoided in pregnancy include rubella, varicella (chickenpox), *Chlamydia*, *Brucella* and *Toxoplasma*. Again, risk assessment and avoidance of hazardous working are essential, and this is a managerial and legal requirement.

Pregnancy may be associated with cultural and emotional pressures, and although in general most pregnant women are physically able and happy to work until the later stages of pregnancy, reassurance may be needed in relation to particular jobs and types of workplace exposure.

More detailed case histories, and examples of sources of support for rehabilitation, can be found in Chapter 8.

REFERENCE

1 Department of Health. *Food Handlers: fitness to work.* London: Department of Health; 1995.

CHAPTER 7

Who else is involved, what do they do, and how can you engage them?

HEALTH AND SAFETY PROFESSIONALS

Occupational physician

The role and responsibilities of occupational physicians are very different from those of the general practitioner or other hospital specialist.

Table 7.1 Comparison of roles and responsibilities

FUNCTION	GENERAL PRACTITIONER	OCCUPATIONAL PHYSICIAN
Diagnosing disease	A major component of day-to-day activity	Not a priority. Discovery of a previously undiagnosed medical condition will lead to communication with the patient's GP
Treating disease or ill health	A major component of day-to-day activity	(Usually) no place for occupational health in treating disease or ill health, but the occupational physician may suggest treatments or strategies that minimise the impact on economic activity
Referral to secondary care	A major responsibility	(Usually) no place for referral except in consultation with the GP, or in an emergency

(cont.)

FUNCTION	GENERAL PRACTITIONER	OCCUPATIONAL PHYSICIAN
Assessing and monitoring response to treatment	Usually the GP's responsibility (often in conjunction with secondary care)	Occupational health departments may be able to help with routine monitoring of health conditions, especially those with a particular potential impact on work (e.g. hypertension, diabetes, bipolar disease)
'Routine' health screening	Integral part of the GP's role	May have a place in occupational health practice, but health screening is usually targeted at specific areas (see below)
Patient advocacy	The GP often acts as the patient's advocate, with Government departments, local authorities, social services and other healthcare organisations	The occupational physician aims to remain impartial – not taking sides with patient, employer, trade union, etc. – and therefore usually avoids advocacy
Advising on state benefits	Significant role	Significant role, particularly where disability is affecting earning capacity
Advising on other sources of help and advice	Significant role	Significant role, particularly agencies that can assist in maintaining employment
Advising on fitness for work	A fundamental, if controversial role	Primary function – related to the individual's usual job and to any alternative jobs
Advising on early retirement due to ill health	May advise a patient to consider early retirement and provide factual information, but usually has no decision-making role	Advises patients on ill health retirement, and often advises pension fund trustees on a patient's eligibility under the rules of the scheme. Sometimes has to advise pension fund 'independently' of the occupational health role for the employer
Health promotion	A fundamental role	A growing role in relation to the 'healthy workplace'

Occupational physicians are primarily involved in preventing ill health from arising at work, assessing fitness for work, and promoting the physical and psychological well-being of staff. Consultations usually have diagnostic and advisory components, but it is fairly unusual for an occupational physician to discover an undiagnosed medical condition. Confirming and assessing what is already known is the usual situation. Communicating with general practitioners and hospital specialists who are responsible for disease management is a key part of that assessment.

The occupational physician is usually employed by (or contracted to) an employer. This relationship can lead to confusion, and sometimes to suspicion as to whether the occupational physician is really an independent medical adviser. The ethics of occupational health practice[1] are clear enough in relation to professional independence and impartiality, but these issues often need to be explained to managers and to patients. One of the areas that regularly causes difficulty is that of patient advocacy. An employee may expect the occupational physician to take their side against managers in situations where there is some interpersonal or managerial dispute. Occupational physicians have to tread a careful line in giving impartial and factual advice, and in some circumstances the occupational health service may appear to be or even risks straying into patient advocacy where injustice (based on a misinterpretation of medical facts) seems possible.

Although it is not strictly necessary to posses a higher qualification in occupational medicine in order to practise as an occupational physician, most employers now look for some evidence of training in the specialty, and may find an unqualified opinion difficult to defend in court, especially if the physician is lacking in experience. For the individual practitioner, the achievement of a formal qualification also provides some practical structure for understanding the need for objectivity in the assessment of employees as compared with clinical practice. The Faculty of Occupational Medicine awards a Diploma (DOccMed) to non-specialists who have undertaken a course of study and passed an examination – usually GPs, but sometimes other specialists whose work may impact on employment issues. Doctors who are pursuing a specialist career, or who wish to study occupational medicine in more depth, will take the examination for the Associateship of the Faculty of Occupational Medicine (AFOM), and may combine this with the 4 years of specialist training and submission of a dissertation which are necessary to achieve full specialist accreditation and become titled a 'Consultant.' Doctors whose role encompasses assessing those who are economically inactive may take the Diploma in Disability Assessment Medicine (DDAM), which is orientated towards making assessments for insurers or for social security purposes. Further information on these qualifications should be obtained from the Faculty, as the structure of specialist training is changing rapidly, and the range of qualifications in occupational medicine is likely to change over the next few years.

Occupational health nurse adviser

Occupational health nurses (also known as occupational health practitioners or advisers) are registered general nurses with a higher qualification in occupational health nursing. Older qualifications such as the Occupational Health Nursing Certificate (OHNC) and the Occupational Health Nursing Diploma (OHND) have been replaced by degree courses, usually associated with community health, and usually leading to qualification as a *specialist practitioner*, which is the nursing equivalent of an accredited specialist doctor. Nurse consultants are still rare, but the shortage of qualified occupational physicians means that this role is becoming increasingly important in the delivery of occupational health services. Nurses may provide the professional lead to an occupational health service. They will provide day-to-day management of the service, immediate care and advice, administration of vaccinations and medications, first-line investigation of cases of ill health in the workplace, workplace environmental visits, and so on. The nurse is likely to be the first point of contact for employees, managers and other health professionals, and is increasingly likely to be involved in managing sickness absence.

Occupational hygienist

Some larger organisations may employ an occupational hygienist (often a chemist or engineer with specialist training) to assess the level of risk in the working environment and to give advice on reducing risk, or on improving the environment. The hygienist will be able to measure levels of fumes, noise, light, dust, etc., and will advise on methods of eliminating or reducing the problem. Specialist occupational hygienists with expertise in dealing with ionising radiation (health physicists) are employed in the nuclear industry. Smaller organisations may use contractors to measure the level of hazard in particular circumstances.

Hygienists use a variety of measuring tools, including light and noise meters, and a range of sampling devices for gases, vapours, fumes and dusts. Measuring general environmental levels of hazard may be important, but hygienists are often asked to measure exposure of individual workers or groups of workers. Assessment of exposure is a vital part of the investigation of occupational ill health.

Safety officer

Most organisations will have designated safety officers, who are trained to interpret health and safety legislation, identify hazards in the workplace and advise on general matters of safety. Their work will often overlap with that of an occupational hygienist, and sometimes with that of the occupational health nurse.

Safety officers come from a variety of backgrounds, often from a science or engineering profession relevant to their employment, and sometimes from the enforcement agencies (e.g. Health and Safety Executive or local authority). Others may come through a trade-union route, perhaps starting as workplace representatives and subsequently acquiring further training. They will usually have a recognised qualification in health and safety, and membership of a professional body such as the Institute of Occupational Safety and Health.

A GP can contact an employer's safety department (where there is one) directly, or may consider raising matters of concern through the occupational health service.

Counsellor

Counselling is widely available in the workplace, often by means of externally commissioned employee assistance programmes (EAPs), commonly delivered by telephone. Workplace counsellors see clients at their own request in privacy, and explore difficulties and other issues, such as distress, life dissatisfaction, or loss of direction and purpose. Through attentive listening, counsellors help their clients to see things more clearly, possibly from a different perspective, thereby enabling choice or change or reducing confusion. Clients are not given advice or direction or judged, but they are helped to explore their life and feelings, and thus to gain an understanding of their anger, anxiety, grief and embarrassment. The counsellor may help the client to examine in detail their behaviour or situations which are proving troublesome, and to find an area where it would be possible to initiate some change as a start and consider the options facing them. As a GP, you may find that a client can access counselling at the workplace more easily and quickly than via the NHS (and without cost to the primary care trust or practice!). In addition, a workplace counsellor will probably understand the context of the employee's job. However, their professional ethics usually mean that they will not communicate directly with occupational health staff. When a patient has suffered an extremely traumatic experience, there is some evidence that a more intense form of talking therapy than directive counselling, perhaps administered by a clinical psychologist, may be necessary.

Occupational psychologist

An occupational psychologist applies psychological knowledge, theory and practice to work in its widest sense. They focus on how work tasks and the conditions of work can affect people, and how people and their characteristics determine what and how work is done. The British Psychological Society defines the work of occupational psychologists as being categorized into eight key areas:

❯ human–machine interaction
❯ design of environments and work – that is, health and safety
❯ personnel selection and assessment, including test and exercise design
❯ performance appraisal and career development
❯ counselling and personal development
❯ training (identification of needs, training design and evaluation)
❯ employee relationships and motivation
❯ organisational development and change.

Work in the area of organisational development includes advising on new technologies such as e-learning, portfolio working and virtual teamworking, helping people to develop leadership, teamwork and communication skills, and advising on employee relationships and schemes to motivate staff.

Involvement in ergonomics and health and safety includes working with engineers, physiologists and ergonomists to improve the design of the working environment and equipment for human users, improving employers' health and safety performance by studying the causes of accidents and their prevention, designing and applying behavioural change interventions, and assessing safety culture and advising on stress prevention and stress management initiatives.

Occupational therapist

Occupational therapists help people to improve their ability to perform tasks at home and at work. These are tasks that are usually taken for granted until there is a health problem that affects a person's ability to do them. Occupational therapists work with individuals who have conditions that are mentally, physically, developmentally or emotionally disabling.

In the workplace, this may involve helping people to develop or adapt motor skills, and may involve input to the ergonomic design or the introduction of aids into the workplace. Occupational therapists with a particular interest in return to work may be members of the Occupational Therapists in Work Practice and Productivity (OTWPP) subsection of their specialist body, the College of Occupational Therapy (COT).

Other specific input from occupational therapists may include cognitive–behavioural therapy (CBT), a directive form of counselling aimed at helping an individual to recognise and respond to the psychological barriers which may be restraining their return to full function, including that at work. Professionals from a range of backgrounds, including nurses and occupational therapists, can be trained to deliver it for the simpler causes, or it can be undertaken via a computerised package such as *Beating the Blues*. CBT can help individuals to improve their functioning by improving their coping with a range of physical and mental disabilities, but it does not deal with the underlying cause, be that an impairment or a work conflict.

Case manager

Case managers are practitioners, usually with a background in healthcare (commonly occupational therapists), who work closely with the individual to coordinate the actions necessary and provide support for them to return to work. The role is a relatively new one, and was developed initially in the insurance industry. Case managers may be members of the Case Management Society UK.

Disability employment advisers and personal advisers: 'Access to Work' and 'Pathways to Work'

It is still unusual for an employer to have direct access to occupational therapists (even in the NHS), but the Regional Disability 'Access to Work' team has occupational therapy expertise. The individual has to request assessment by 'Access to Work' by visiting the Job Centre, which will normally arrange an interview with the Disability Employment Adviser (DEA). A DEA is a Job Centre Officer with special experience and training in responding to the employment needs of people with disabilities. It may also be possible to obtain access to occupational therapists through the Condition Management Programmes (CMP) run by the Department for Work and Pensions through the various 'Pathways to Work' schemes in most parts of the UK. CMP can be offered to individuals in receipt of Incapacity Benefit following a referral from a work-focused interview (WFI) at the Job Centre to a personal adviser. Personal advisers are Job Centre Officers who have been specially trained to work with people who have long-term illnesses, rather than disabilities.

Physiotherapist

Some larger organisations have recognised the benefits of employing physio-therapists to assess and treat musculoskeletal problems in employees, or to provide expertise in the area of ergonomic design of work tasks. This is particularly true in organisations where musculoskeletal demand and residual risk of injury are significant. Important aspects of physiotherapy in industry include predicting what tasks may result in musculoskeletal injury from misuse or overuse, advising on reducing risk, and treating injury early. NHS waiting times for routine physiotherapy treatment can be long, and early intervention to assess and treat back pain, shoulder pain, neck problems, etc. often enables an early return to work. Unfortunately, access to physiotherapy at work is still very limited. Where physiotherapy is available, triaging can be used to manage the resource cost-effectively. Commonly the employer funds five or six sessions, with the first session being used for treatment planning. Physiotherapists with a special interest in occupational health may belong to the Association of Chartered Physiotherapists in Occupational Health and Ergonomics (ACPOHE), a specialist subgroup of the Chartered Society of Physiotherapy.

Ergonomist

Ergonomics is about using knowledge of human abilities and limitations to design and build for comfort, efficiency, productivity and safety. It is the application of scientific information concerning humans to the design of objects, systems and environment for human use. Ergonomics is implicated in everything which involves people. Well-designed work systems should always embody ergonomic principles.

Large organisations may employ ergonomists, particularly where the interaction between the human employee and machines or equipment is critical to productivity. When problems arise (e.g. musculoskeletal strain or injury, psychological stress, excessive fatigue), an employer may either seek the advice of their in-house ergonomists, or engage consultants.

Physiotherapists, safety professionals, and occupational physicians and nurses all have some training in ergonomic principles, but where complex interactions between humans and machines are taking place, or where new processes are being designed, the advice of a professional ergonomist can be essential in order to avert future health and safety problems.

ORGANISATIONAL SUPPORT

Line manager

If an employee is struggling to maintain their attendance or performance at work because of ill health or injury, the line manager will be the first person to notice this, and will have a responsibility to investigate and intervene. In an ideal world, the line manager is therefore the best person to provide initial support and encouragement when enabling someone to return to work or to remain at work against a background of health problems.

In practice, of course, employees may not always have an open, friendly and trusting relationship with their line manager, and relationships may be strained further if the employee is off sick or not performing very well.

Line managers have a key responsibility to identify precisely what tasks an employee is expected to perform at work, which tasks are crucial and which can be given to other people or avoided altogether, what hours of work or shift patterns are necessary in the job, and what level of productivity is critical to the business. Ultimately, an employer has a right to expect a certain level of attendance and performance or productivity, and defining that level in relation to an employee's health is likely to be the line manager's responsibility. Thus line managers need to communicate carefully with the individual, and with occupational health and safety advisers. This is easier said than done if interpersonal relationships between managers and employees are strained, and it is not unusual for occupational health and safety or human resource managers to have to facilitate meetings and advise on reasonable ways forward.

Line managers often struggle to maintain contact with employees who are off sick. They may be concerned that any attempted contact with an employee will be seen as harassment. Employees may resent being contacted by their manager when they are 'off sick', and view this as intrusion into a legitimate medical situation. Most employers expect their employees to accept and maintain some level of contact with their managers beyond simply submitting sick notes.

The key to all this is for managers to maintain good relationships and good communication with their staff at all times, so that if an employee does need to be off sick due to illness or injury, maintaining friendly contact is easy and leads automatically to non-threatening discussion about resettlement at work.

There is nothing to stop the GP making direct contact with a patient's line manager, particularly if the GP is uncertain about precisely what tasks the individual is required to carry out at work. Having said that, line managers may press a GP for inappropriate medical information about an employee, and communication about rehabilitation, the effects of illness or injury and capacity for work is usually best channelled through occupational health professionals.

Human resources

The conventional view of human resources activity centres around hiring and firing. However, human resource managers are more closely involved in giving advice to general managers on employment law, good practice and developing individuals' skills and careers. Human resource departments may have dedicated sections for training and development, and are clearly key players when an individual employee needs to change career or job due to ill health or injury. Human resource managers are also usually involved in disputes between employees and managers, most commonly in the role of advisers (putting in place mediation, etc.). These are areas where human resources and occupational health practice overlap, and where general practitioners may be asked to give factual information about the health of their patients. It is important that such reports are commissioned and interpreted via occupational health, as consent given for a report to be sent directly to human resources officials or line managers might not be regarded in law as freely given, and interpreting the terms or language of the outside practitioner would usually benefit from occupational health input. Human resource managers may form a useful source of reference or support for employees who feel unable to approach their line manager.

Trade-union representative

The role of the trade-union representative in any health situation will depend very much on the nature of the relationship between the employee and the employer. In straightforward cases of ill health or injury, where communication between line managers, human resource departments and the employee is good, the trade-union representative may not need to get involved.

In other situations, the employee may need the advocacy skills of a trade-union representative to assist negotiations about the return to work. Trade unions may have other specific roles in situations where illness or injury has been caused by work, and measures need to be taken to investigate risks in the workplace and to reduce the risk to other employees.

Employees may benefit from the presence of the trade-union representative during discussions with their line manager about their sickness absence and their plans to return to work. Occasionally, employees will bring their trade-union representative to consultations with an occupational physician or an occupational health nurse. This may imply that the employee believes the occupational health service is acting on behalf of the employer, and that the employee therefore needs advocacy support in dealing with the occupational health service. Employees and trade-union representatives can usually be reassured about impartiality, and so long as the employee does not mind discussing their health concerns openly and fully in front of their trade-union representative, occupational health services are usually quite relaxed about this. It is better that all of the parties concerned understand in some detail the nature of the functional restrictions that illness or injury may cause, and can contribute to plans for overcoming those restrictions and returning the employee to work.

Trade-union representatives can also provide much less formalised support, such as keeping in touch with sick or disabled employees in or out of work, ensuring the applicability of reasonable adjustments, interpreting pensions regulations, and simple tasks such as walking/driving into work with a newly returned employee to boost their confidence.

Occupational health project adviser

A number of UK cities, including Liverpool, Sheffield, Leeds and Bradford, benefit from the activity of occupational health charities whose role is to provide advocacy to employees who have health problems caused by or troubling them at work. Each project is slightly different, but they share a common approach to working with individuals in an advocacy role, usually through lay advisers who are trained and experienced in case management or health and safety. Chapter 5 is written by such an adviser. Sometimes the advocacy service is delivered on the premises of GPs. These charities do not provide mainstream occupational health services, but do pioneer innovation in occupational health practice.

Benefits adviser

Many local authorities provide benefits advice, often described as 'welfare rights', as do some voluntary organisations (e.g. the Citizens Advice Bureaux). Such advice tends to be based around the short-term needs and expectations of the individual (e.g. for Housing Benefit), and its urgent nature may lead to overlooking the longer-term health benefits of sustained employment in a healthy setting.

GP employment adviser

In a number of parts of the UK, experiments are taking place in which employment professionals, frequently seconded from Job Centres, are working in some GP practices to help to return long-term sick individuals to employment, or to prevent employees who have recently gone off sick from losing contact with the workplace.

REFERENCE

1 Faculty of Occupational Medicine. *Guidance on Ethics for Occupational Physicians.* 6th ed. London: Faculty of Occupational Medicine; 2006.

CHAPTER 8

Specific causes of absence: case discussions

In this chapter we shall look at some common causes of absence from work, how they may present to the general practitioner, an occupational health view, and some suggestions on how these conditions and problems may be tackled.

CASE 1: 'STRESS'

John is a 42-year-old project engineer with a large aerospace company. You haven't seen much of him over the years; the last consultation was 6 years ago when he injured his knee playing squash. He appears reluctant to talk to you and apologises for bothering you, but it quickly becomes apparent that he is anxious and rather distressed.

When pressed, John admits that he hasn't been sleeping very well, hates going to work and doesn't understand why he feels so 'bad.' He has lost interest in social activities, and his wife has complained that he is miserable at home.

He finds it difficult to get off to sleep, he is worrying about aspects of his job, and he wakes up early thinking about tasks he hasn't completed. He is living off bars of chocolate at work, and is drinking more alcohol than usual.

When you ask him why he thinks he has become like this, the only explanation he can offer is that the project in which he is involved at work hasn't been going well, his line manager is pushing him all the time to solve problems, and he feels he has little support from junior colleagues. The only other possible cause is some anxiety about his 15-year-old son, who does not appear to be taking schoolwork very seriously.

What is the diagnosis? How would you assess the severity of the symptoms and decide on a diagnostic label?

With symptoms like these, mild anxiety/depression seems to be the most likely diagnosis. Alternatively, this could be described as work-related stress. In conventional medical terms the general practitioner will need to consider 'treatment.' There may be a place for antidepressants, and there may also be a place for 'counselling', if the GP has access to this.

One of the key questions at this stage is whether giving John a sick note – authorising him to take time off work – will be appropriate and useful.

It may be that his symptoms are significant enough for you to want him to stay away from work for a while. Part of the difficult that the GP faces (in what may be a short consultation) is getting a feel for how psychologically 'hazardous' the workplace is for John at present. Some time off work may help John to get his anxieties back into perspective, but equally the problems may still be there when he goes back, and he may have an even more overflowing 'in tray.'

If John works for a large company, the chances are that he will have an occupational health service. If he hasn't already contacted his occupational health department, you could certainly suggest that he does so, as a 'self-referral.' The occupational health department has several advantages over the GP in this situation. They may already know that John's department is something of a 'hot spot' for stress at present. It may therefore not come as a surprise to them that John is suffering from symptoms of stress. The occupational health department may also have some insight into the specific causes of stress in that department, or could investigate why John may be suffering from excessive pressure.

Getting John back to work

The barriers

> John's symptoms, his understanding of his condition, his views on the causes (yellow flags), his attitudes to his work, his colleagues and his employer (blue flags), and his concerns about the future.
> The availability of support services, including counselling and occupational health support.
> The stigma of 'mental illness' – for John, his colleagues and his employer.
> The work environment. Will it be just as stressful when he returns?
> The GP's attitudes and beliefs. Is John's GP positive about helping him to return to work? Does the GP believe that work is intrinsically good or intrinsically bad for health?

> The employer's attitude to assisting and facilitating a return to work. Does the employer believe that John must feel '100 per cent' before he should go back to work?
> Financial pressures or constraints (black flags), including sick pay and insurance payments (e.g. mortgage protection policies).

Overcoming the barriers

THE GP'S ROLE

As John's GP, you can offer conventional medical advice and you should consider whether advising him to stay away from work is appropriate. You need to avoid a situation where John is off for so long that he loses his confidence, and starts to worry more about the backlog of work, and what his colleagues are saying and thinking about the situation.

As a GP you cannot influence the nature of the stresses at work. If there is an occupational health service, and you have the time and John's consent, you could make contact with an occupational health nurse or physician to raise your concerns about the workplace.

Minimising time lost from work is important, but returning to work too soon and having to go off sick again because the pressures are still too great is not helpful.

Is an antidepressant appropriate? If the somatic and psychological symptoms are sufficiently worrying, an antidepressant with some anxiolytic activity may be appropriate, but patients such as John are often reluctant to take them.

COUNSELLING

Counselling or other forms of psychotherapeutic support would be useful here – and probably as useful in the long term as an antidepressant. John will feel better if he can explain his fears and feelings to someone who is skilled in reflective listening, or in solution-focused brief therapy. Perhaps formal cognitive–behavioural therapy (CBT) would be helpful in the longer term, but some people with acute anxiety/depression find it hard to engage with CBT while they are still distressed.

Accessing CBT through the NHS can be difficult. Indeed, accessing any help from trained psychotherapists can take months – time that we really don't have if we are to help John back to work quickly. Some employers have counselling services, but they vary from telephone helplines (hardly the kind of support that John would need) to competent clinical psychology.

There is still a huge stigma associated with any mental health problem, and people are often embarrassed to be off work with 'stress', particularly if they are in professional jobs. They view absence as 'weakness.' Counsellors can work with the GP and the occupational health service to help John to understand the nature of his illness and to overcome any sense of embarrassment he may have.

THE OCCUPATIONAL HEALTH SERVICE ROLE

The occupational health service will be helping management to look at the sources of stress (a risk assessment), with the aim of tackling the main causes. There is little point in John taking time off work if he goes back to an uncontrolled psychological 'hazard.'

The Health and Safety Executive defines causes of occupational stress in terms of control, relationships, role, demands, change and support. If John's working relationships are poor, he is getting little support, the demands of the job are overwhelming, and the project he is involved with is running into problems that he cannot control, there are good reasons for him to be experiencing symptoms of stress.

The principal role of the occupational health service in this situation is to try to assess John's emotional health and his capacity to cope with work demands, against the backdrop of what they know about the organisation and the current work environment.

The initial return to work

Timing the return to work in this situation is something of an art, and a direct discussion between the GP (who knows the individual's health and personality) and the occupational health department (who know the work environment and support mechanisms) is likely to lead to the best and most appropriate timing for resettlement.

Keeping in touch

John needs to be encouraged to maintain or restore contact with his line manager and his colleagues. This is often difficult because of the problem of 'stigma.' However, early informal contacts are very helpful. John could be encouraged to meet colleagues on 'neutral territory' – perhaps for a coffee. There is a tendency for colleagues to be less than encouraging with regard to return to work. We often hear remarks like 'Oh, you don't want to come back yet – it's complete chaos in there!'

Phased return

The occupational health service will usually advise managers and individuals on a plan of 'phased' return to work. There isn't much science in this. It is usually a matter of assessing the balance between what we feel an individual can cope with, what tasks may be given to them when they return to work, and not being averse to building up attendance at work reasonably quickly. Prolonged, slow increases in hours of work that take place over more than 4 or 5 weeks are rarely appropriate. Alongside reduced hours of work, John will need to be given confidence-building tasks in the first few days after his return. Being faced with an intimidating and overloaded in tray and not knowing where to start is unlikely to result in a successful and sustained resettlement. However, being encouraged by colleagues or line managers to pick up and complete some straightforward tasks will help to build up confidence. The occupational health service often needs to remind managers of this simple truth.

Financial issues

One of the barriers to a phased return to work at this stage may be financial. On the one hand, John may have company sick pay (often full pay for several months, followed by half pay), but if he returns to work on reduced hours, his employer may insist that he uses holiday entitlement to reduce his hours, or that he is only paid for the number of hours that he works. There is obviously no incentive for John to reduce his hours for very long if he is being penalised in this way. There is little that the GP or the occupational health service can do to influence company policy, other than to point out to the employer the advantages of helping John back to work and not penalising a phased resettlement.

Other financial disincentives to attempting an early return to work include mortgage or credit card payment insurance policies that have a 'waiting period.' Some policies require an individual to have been off work for more than a month before they will cover mortgage payments. If John returns to work but can't cope, and has to go off sick again, he may have to wait before his mortgage or credit card protection policy will pay again. He may therefore want to be absolutely certain in his own mind that he won't 'fail' and suffer financially.

Continuing support

The first hurdle is to get John back into the workplace and talking to his colleagues. Once he is doing elements of his normal job, he may well find that his confidence returns quickly. It makes sense for the occupational health service to see him regularly (perhaps every couple of weeks), just briefly, in the first couple of months after his return. The nurse or doctor can then pick up any clues about relapsing anxiety or inappropriate environmental pressures.

Managers sometimes ask whether employees in John's situation are 'disabled' within the meaning of the Disability Discrimination Act. If John's symptoms have lasted or are likely to last for more than 12 months, and if – during that time – his normal day-to-day activities have been substantially impaired (e.g. he is unable to go out shopping or socialise normally), this may be regarded by an Employment Tribunal as a disability.

CASE 2: 'BACK PAIN'

Marion is a 36-year-old healthcare assistant. She has consulted you four times in the past 3 years because of back pain. On each occasion, you have prescribed non-steroidal anti-inflammatory medication and analgesia. She consults you again complaining of low backache radiating to her buttocks, which is made worse by stooping. She is overweight, but has no other medical problems.

Basically, Marion wants time off work. She tells you that her job is 'heavy', working on an acute medical ward where many of the patients are elderly and need hands-on nursing care and assistance with bodily functions.

What clinical criteria do you take into account when deciding what the underlying pathology might be and whether further investigations might be justified?
Assessing Marion for 'red flags' is most important. These include:
- age of onset < 20 or > 55 years
- violent trauma (fall from a height, road traffic accident)
- constant, progressive, non-mechanical pain
- thoracic pain
- past medical history of carcinoma, systemic steroids, HIV or drug abuse
- systemically unwell (fever, unexplained weight loss)
- structural deformity, persistent severe restriction of lumbar flexion
- widespread neurological signs or symptoms
- cauda equina syndrome.

Getting Marion back to work
The barriers
- Marion's symptoms, her beliefs and fears, her understanding of the nature of back pain (yellow flags), and her relationships with her manager and colleagues (blue flags).
- Marion's mood and the possibility of low-grade depression (orange flag).

❯ The availability of physiotherapy and other quick treatment options.
❯ The likelihood of short-term or long-term adjustments to her work.
❯ The GP's understanding of back pain, and their commitment to encouraging a return to work.
❯ The employer's beliefs about back pain, and their commitment to assisting resettlement where someone isn't '100 per cent' symptom-free.
  The presence of 'flags' suggests a risk of chronicity and illness behaviour.

Overcoming the barriers

THE GP'S ROLE

If you decide that Marion's problem is simple mechanical back pain, how will you manage it in the short term?

There is plenty of guidance from the Royal College of General Practitioners and the Faculty of Occupational Medicine (*see* Further reading section at the end of this chapter) on managing back pain, but the key is to manage Marion's pain with simple analgesics and non-steroidal anti-inflammatory drugs, to encourage her to remain mobile and – if at all possible – to arrange some physical treatment.

You may need to explore Marion's attitudes to work and her beliefs about her back pain. There is a good case for referring her to a counsellor or physiotherapist with special expertise in assessing and modifying the psycho-social aspects of back pain, if one is available to you. It is most important not to reinforce Marion's beliefs that work is inherently bad or damaging, or that she will do herself real damage if she returns to work, or even tries to keep mobile.

As Marion works in the health service, it may be possible to arrange physio-therapy or even assessment in a spinal triage clinic quickly, either through direct contact with the physiotherapy department or via the occupational health service.

THE PHYSIOTHERAPIST'S ROLE

As well as offering assessment, physical interventions and exercise training, the physiotherapist may be able to help with retraining Marion in moving and handling techniques. There is likely to be a moving and handling coordinator in Marion's workplace, and training may be shared with the physiotherapy department.

THE OCCUPATIONAL HEALTH SERVICE ROLE

The occupational health service needs to know about Marion's problem as soon as possible. Whether her manager refers her formally to the occupational health service for advice and an opinion on her fitness for work will depend very much on local policies and procedures. It is therefore important that either Marion self-refers, or the GP contacts the occupational health service. Occupational health professionals may be able to facilitate physiotherapy, and will be able to start a discussion with Marion and her line managers about the resettlement process. If there are particular workplace problems (e.g. a need for moving and handling training, or a lack of moving and handling equipment), the occupational health service may be able to investigate and intervene.

The initial return to work

Once Marion is mobile and her pain is reasonably controlled, her GP and the occupational health service should be encouraging her to think about returning to work. If her negative beliefs are to be overcome, she will need to be confident that her ward manager will modify her moving and handling duties on her return to work, at least in the initial stages, and that her return will be supported. The occupational health service will be working with the line manager to help to overcome any attitude barriers within the organisation. Unfortunately, it is still common for managers not to want a member of staff back at work unless they are perceived to be '100 per cent' fit, and to regard any back pain in a nurse as a major barrier to continuing employment.

It makes sense for Marion to reduce her working hours for a few shifts, as she learns to become mobile again in the workplace. Standing, stooping and bending at work are all rather different to being at home.

As with the case of John (see above), there may be financial barriers (black flags) associated with Marion's return to work. She may be penalised by being asked to use holiday entitlement or lose money if she temporarily reduces her hours.

Continued support

There is a role for the occupational health service in talking to Marion occasionally, to encourage her to continue with her back exercises and to look positively at her nursing career. Clearly, if her back pain recurs and becomes significantly disabling in relation to her 'manual' job, redeployment will need to be considered.

CASE 3: 'EPILEPSY'

Brian is a 26-year-old instrument technician who works in a power station. He suffers from epilepsy; he had complex partial seizures in his teenage years and was put on phenytoin. He was recently advised to change his medication to sodium valproate. Unfortunately, this change of medication led to him suffering two seizures at home, and significant sedation and short-term memory loss. His neurologist is now reducing his valproate and adding levetiracetam.

He has been off work for 6 weeks, since he had a seizure. He wants to return to work, but is not sure whether he could cope at present because of his memory problems.

Brian is normally a very fit man, training hard and running marathons, but he has been advised by his neurologist to stop running for the moment. He finds all the advice confusing.

Getting Brian back to work

The barriers

- Brian's anxiety about whether he will have another fit and whether he is sufficiently alert to do his job.
- The real risk of him having another fit at work.
- The employer's attitude to Brian's safety and the safety of those around him.
- The 'medical' anxiety about him returning to work (including the anxiety of his neurologist and GP), together with potentially conflicting advice.

Overcoming the barriers

THE GP'S ROLE

As his GP, your main role must be to reassure Brian and to interpret the advice that the neurologist is giving him. Whether or not it is safe for him to go back to work is probably an occupational health and managerial decision rather than one that a GP can make easily. You may not have detailed knowledge of his workplace, or even a detailed understanding of the tasks that he undertakes at work, so advising on fitness for work in a situation like this can be very difficult for you as his GP.

THE NEUROLOGIST AND SPECIALIST NURSE PRACTITIONER

Although the neurologist can give specialist technical advice on medication and controlling seizures, they may not be in any better a position than you as his GP to give advice on fitness for work. Indeed, there is a real risk in this kind of situation that Brian will be given conflicting or inadequate advice in a busy clinic. A specialist epilepsy nurse may be a good source of practical and sensible advice, particularly in relation to issues like physical exercise. Why should Brian stop his training at the moment? Is it just in case he has a seizure while out running, or are there other clinical reasons? The specialist nurse can interpret and clarify the advice that Brian has been given.

THE OCCUPATIONAL HEALTH SERVICE

The occupational health nurse or physician will have a very good idea of precisely what tasks Brian undertakes at work. It is likely that his history of epilepsy will be known to the occupational health service, and that some modifications to his job will already have been in place. For example, it is likely that he will not be required to climb ladders or work on unguarded heights or moving machinery. Any tools that he uses should be assessed for safety (e.g. they should shut down automatically if he loses consciousness while using them). Depending on the precise nature of his job, he may have been restricted from working alone. All of these modifications to his job would already have been advised by the occupational health service as part of good occupational health practice and the requirements of the Disability Discrimination Act.

The occupational health team will therefore want to talk to Brian again about the changes in his medical condition, particularly any sedation or problems with cognitive function. The question will again be one of his safety and the safety of those with whom he works. Liaison with a specialist epilepsy nurse would be most helpful.

The initial return to work

Overcoming Brian's anxieties will be important, and the occupational health service will need to assess the likelihood of his having a seizure at work. If his work has been modified previously, it is likely that his line manager and at least some of his work colleagues will know of his medical condition. If they don't, the occupational health team would encourage Brian to think about telling them – and also any first aiders – about his condition. We can't make him tell people about his epilepsy, but we can encourage him to be open so that people around him are not too shocked if he has a seizure while at work.

Regaining his confidence on returning to work will be important, and it may be sensible for him to restrict his activities to 'workshop' tasks for a month or so, to assess whether his memory and motor skills are intact, and to avoid him going out and about in the power station until he is reasonably confident that his medication is effective. In the early stages of a change in medication, shift work may well be contraindicated, to avoid any risk of sleep deprivation or altering the timing of medication affecting his condition.

The occupational health team can explain these issues to his managers – perhaps in a meeting between Brian and his line manager. Brian may want his trade union to know about his problems and to be involved in any meetings with management.

Continuing support

Much will depend on Brian remaining free of seizures in the future. If he continues to have seizures at regular intervals, or has problems with sedation or altered mood due to his medication, more permanent restrictions on his activities may be necessary. This would be unfortunate, but a good employer would listen to the advice of the occupational health service.

Note that in this case, which is about fitness to return to work, the 'flags' are not relevant.

CASE 4: 'CANCER'

Rose is 52 years old, and works part-time as a catering assistant at a local college. Three months ago she was diagnosed with carcinoma in her right breast. She had a lumpectomy and axillary clearance, and is now undergoing chemotherapy. She will have radiotherapy when the chemotherapy has finished. She has been told that the prognosis is 'good', as just a single lymph node was affected.

She is worried about returning to work, and can't decide whether she wants to try, or whether she just won't be able to cope. At the moment her cycles of chemotherapy are making her feel quite ill. She is also worried about her financial situation if she can't get back to work.

Getting Rose back to work

The barriers

❭ Rose's mood and confidence. Will she have any lasting psychological issues relating to her diagnosis and treatment?
❭ Her physical limitations. She is right-handed, so will she have any problems reaching, lifting and carrying with her right arm? Will she have any lymphoedema?
❭ How tired will she be at the end of her course of chemotherapy and radiotherapy?
❭ What will be her employer's attitude to keeping her job open?

Overcoming the barriers

THE GP'S ROLE

Again this is very much about maintaining a positive approach to the subject of work, while acknowledging that there may be some long-lasting psychological issues as well as some physical constraints.

As GPs we often feel – quite understandably – that we wish to be guided by the patient in a situation like this, and we may want to acquiesce to any line that the patient takes, whether that is to return to work quickly or (at the other extreme) to 'retire.' Emphasising the importance of work, and the fact that once Rose has come through the physical and emotional pressures of chemotherapy and radiotherapy she should be able to manage her part-time job, will be important. Keeping the options open for a return to work once she has recovered may be important for the psychological aspects of her health as well as the financial ones.

THE BREAST CARE NURSE

Most oncology centres will have a breast care nurse who can keep in touch with patients like Rose throughout their treatment. In this situation it would be helpful for the breast care nurse to communicate with both the GP and the occupational health service (if there is one). There is a real danger here of mixed messages confusing Rose. If the breast care nurse or the GP are uneasy about resettlement at work, this will be picked up by Rose and it will affect her confidence.

THE OCCUPATIONAL HEALTH SERVICE

The college should have access to an occupational health service, if not an in-house service. The role of the occupational health service in this situation will be to reinforce the message of work being 'good', and certainly feasible. Some adjustments may be necessary on Rose's return to work. Much will depend on how her right arm is – whether there is any residual immobility in the shoulder, or any lasting lymphoedema. It may be necessary to restrict her lifting and reaching for a while (or perhaps permanently). The occupational health service can assess this more precisely than the GP could in relation to the tasks in the workplace. There may also be some anxiety about injuries to Rose's right hand or arm. For example, oven burns on the right hand or wrist which have become infected may cause problems with the altered lymphatic drainage.

If Rose raises the possibility of retirement due to ill health, the occupational health service is probably in a better position to assess whether this is appropriate or likely to succeed than is the GP (who may feel instinctively that this must be 'best' if Rose wants it). If Rose is in the Local Government Pension Scheme, the criteria that are applied (by an independent qualified occupational physician) will be whether (on the balance of probabilities) Rose would remain unfit to do her substantive job, or a similar job, up to the age of 65 years. If the information about the prognosis changes, or if Rose has a significant and permanent problem with her right arm, retirement may be appropriate. Otherwise, an application would be likely to fail. If Rose aspires to retire, there is a risk of a black flag.

COLLEGE MANAGEMENT

It is most important in a situation like this that college management personnel maintain contact with Rose and (if they can do so) assure her that her job will still be open to her. By definition, as someone who has cancer, she is disabled within the meaning of the Disability Discrimination Act, and one 'reasonable adjustment' may be to accept a prolonged absence from work in relation to her treatment and recovery.

Continuing support

Contact between the occupational health service and college management should ease Rose back to work. In addition to the physical tiredness that she will experience on returning to work, she will face emotional pressures (e.g. from people asking her how she is). Depending on how much contact she has had with colleagues and friends at work during her absence, and how much she wants to talk about her illness, these pressures can be very distressing. The occupational health service would acknowledge them and try to prepare her for them.

CASE 5: 'SURGERY' (A COLOSTOMY)

Pete is 36 years old. He has had ulcerative colitis for many years, constantly struggling with his symptoms and time off work, before finally losing his job as a paint sprayer in a car body shop when his symptoms stopped him attending regularly. Medication never really controlled his symptoms for very long. He ended up having a colostomy 2 months ago, and has now started to feel dramatically better. He is talking about going back to work – either to his old line of work or to something new.

Getting Pete back to work

The barriers

> Pete is well motivated, and now he is feeling better, he wants to work. However, he is concerned about his physical limitations. He is coping with his stoma and bag, but is worried about dealing with it in the workplace. Will it affect his performing physical tasks at work?

> What will be a potential employer's attitude to his problem?

Overcoming the barriers

THE GP'S ROLE

As his GP, encouraging Pete and making sure that he has access to the appropriate specialist advice from a stoma nurse is important. Depending on what his future job might be, different types of bag or equipment might be needed. You may also have to give basic occupational health advice in this situation with regard to what Pete might be able to do, if specialist input is not available.

OCCUPATIONAL HEALTH SERVICE

The problem here is that there is unlikely to be any specialist occupational health input to this situation. If Pete is able to return to his old employer, and if they have access to an occupational health service (perhaps through NHS Plus or the Health and Safety Executive's Workplace Health Direct scheme), they could access that expertise to assess Pete's fitness for work, and any adjustments that might be necessary. Otherwise, his GP may be the only source of medical advice.

JOBCENTRE PLUS

If Pete is looking for a new job, the advice of the Job Centre will be necessary. It may be that he is confident enough to apply for any job that utilises his previous skills, or any job that he wants to try, without discussing with the Job Centre advisers his recent medical problems. If he does want to discuss the suitability of jobs, he would talk to the Disability Employment Adviser.

Continuing support

Pete may need some specific advice on his fitness for work with a colostomy, and this advice would be best coming from an occupational health service. If that isn't possible, the GP needs to bear in mind the following points and be prepared to support Pete with some detailed advocacy.

> Will he be repeatedly lifting and bending? Will this affect his stoma?

❯ Does he need to wear specific personal protective equipment that might affect his stoma or bag? Can he wear appropriate trousers or overalls, so that his bag isn't impeded and he can get to it easily if necessary?
❯ Can he have easy access to a toilet if he needs it?
❯ Is he likely to be working in hot conditions? Will this affect his bag, the adhesive, or even his fluid balance? This is usually only an issue with ileostomies, but it is worth bearing in mind.

In the end, there probably isn't a good reason to stop Pete returning to his old job as a paint sprayer, if he can overcome the anxieties of potential employers.

FURTHER READING

Carter JT, Birrell LN, editors. *Occupational Health Guidelines for the Management of Low Back Pain at Work: principal recommendations.* London: Faculty of Occupational Medicine; 2000.

Royal College of General Practitioners. *Clinical Guidelines for the Management of Acute Low Back Pain.* London: Royal College of General Practitioners; 1996 (Review published in 1998).

CHAPTER 9

The UK social security system and rehabilitation

BACKGROUND

The UK social security system for sickness and disability dates from the social, industrial and medical revolutions of the nineteenth century, prompted in particular by the need to provide for industrial injury. It was recognised that only the state could provide ultimate cover for the traditional risks of occupational injury, sickness, old age and unemployment. Such social insurance improves not only the standard of life of individual workers, but also the economic, social and political stability of society. Over the last century the original concept of *social insurance* has evolved into a broader concept of *social security*, and the focus has shifted from the industrial worker to the citizen per se. 'Incapacity' benefits provide income replacement for people whose capacity for work is limited by sickness and disability. Such benefits raise the question of how to define and identify individuals who are 'incapacitated for work.'

The philosophy of 'work for those who can, security for those who cannot' reflects two broad policy goals:

» *social protection* – to provide adequate income support for people whose capacity for work is limited by sickness or disability; in other words, financial support for individuals, which tend to be regarded as 'passive' policies

» *social integration* – to provide realistic opportunities and support for sick and disabled people who have (some) capacity to work, to enable disabled people to participate as fully as possible in society; in other words, more 'active' policies to support rehabilitation.

Social protection and social integration policies complement each other, but there is an inevitable tension between them. The ideal is to integrate these two approaches as effectively as possible. To resolve the potential conflict, financial support such as that provided by state benefits can be balanced with more positive support into work. Incapacity benefits cannot be considered in isolation, but must be placed in a broader social and political context, including in particular employment and anti-poverty policies and targets.

Over the past 50 years there have been profound economic, social, cultural and political changes in society (*see* Box 9.1), to which social security systems have had to adapt. Social security in the UK is now the largest area of public expenditure, with costs in 2006 exceeding £110 billion per annum.

BOX 9.1   SOCIAL CHANGES SINCE 1948[1]

- Economic prosperity and rising material standards of living.
- The role of women and family structures (in particular, the number of women working, gender equality and lone-parent families).
- Labour-market changes and patterns of work (globalisation, greater flexibility and mobility, more part-time and fixed-contract working, lower job security).
- Overall higher levels of employment, but also higher levels of (male) unemployment (since the 1980s).
- Patterns of retirement (working fewer years but living longer, increased availability of employment pensions, trends towards early retirement).
- Changing attitudes to work, sickness, disability and social security benefits.
- Social (including disability) rights and responsibilities.
- Individual liberty and rising expectations.
- Disenchantment with professional 'authority' and medical 'models.'

WORK AND WORKLESSNESS

Work is a major part of life. It provides the income and rewards to sustain lifestyle, independence and security, a structure for how we spend our lives, and the social contact, relationships and status that help to define the individual and his or her role in society. Participation in work is probably the main route to social inclusion and integration in today's society. Sickness and disability represent threats to a full and happy life, and incapacity for work is one of the most significant impacts on the individual and their family, as well as on employers, the economy and wider society. This impact is partly financial, but is also about broader goals of social inclusion.

Job retention, return to work and reintegration are therefore the most relevant and important (albeit not the only) goals and outcome measures of healthcare, rehabilitation and the social security system, across the range of health problems that cause incapacity. Loss of capacity for work due to sickness and disability is the basis for 'incapacity' benefits. Building capacity, improving functioning and (re-)entering the labour force is the best exit from benefits dependency. Even when disabled people cannot be fully self-supporting, everyone may gain by enabling them to make some contribution.

In the UK, two to three million disabled people already work, and another million economically inactive people with health problems, such as those on state incapacity benefits, say that they would like to work. There is a growing social consensus that sees employment as a desirable form of social participation for all adults, and that is applicable to sick and disabled people as much as to everyone else. At the same time, there is a stigma attached to disability, and particularly to mental illness, which tends to exclude people affected from all aspects of life.

On balance, the evidence shows that work is good for physical and mental health and well-being, while there is strong evidence that worklessness is harmful (*see* Box 9.2).

BOX 9.2 THE BENEFITS OF WORK AND THE HARM CAUSED BY WORKLESSNESS[2]

Work is beneficial for people with sickness or disability, in terms of:	*Long-term worklessness leads to:*
Symptom management	Loss of fitness
Recovery and rehabilitation	Physical and mental deterioration
Self-esteem and confidence	Poor physical and mental health
Self-identity	Psychological distress and depression
'Normalisation' of activities and participation	Increased suicide and mortality rates
Improved social functioning	Loss of work-related attitudes and habits
Quality of life	Poverty
Social inclusion	Social exclusion

Too often, work is seen as the problem, rather than as the goal or part of the solution, and healthcare professionals are as guilty of making this mistake as any other group. The past emphasis on the prevention of occupational injury and disease has led to an assumption that work is potentially 'harmful' to health. However, for many less severe health problems this is contrary to the evidence, namely that an earlier return to work reduces rather than increases the risk of recurrent or persistent trouble. The second assumption is that rest from work is part of treatment. In fact, modern approaches to the management of most common health problems emphasise the importance of continuing ordinary activities as normally as possible, and of early return to work. The third assumption is that it is not possible or advisable to return to work until symptoms are completely 'cured' (i.e. until the patient is '100 per cent' recovered). However, modern clinical and occupational management emphasises that return to work as early as possible is an essential part of treatment for many health problems, even if there are some persistent symptoms. Not only is work the goal and outcome of treatment, but also work itself is therapeutic, aids recovery and is often the best form of rehabilitation. The important caveat to this is that the quality of the work is very important.

ILLNESS, DISABILITY AND INCAPACITY FOR WORK

Words like 'illness', 'disability' and 'sickness' are often used loosely as if they were interchangeable, reflecting lack of clear thinking about fundamental concepts (*see* Box 9.3).

BOX 9.3 THE DISTINCTION BETWEEN KEY TERMS

Disease is objective, medically diagnosed pathology (i.e. it is a disorder of structure or function of the human organism).

Impairment is significant, demonstrable deviation or loss of body structure or function – sometimes referred to a 'loss of faculty.'

Symptoms are bodily or mental sensations that reach consciousness (e.g. aches, pains, fatigue, breathlessness, anxiety).

Illness is the subjective feeling of being unwell (i.e. it is an internal, personal experience).

Disability is limitation of activities and restriction of participation in people with physical and/or mental conditions or impairments.

Sickness (or the 'sick role') is a social status accorded to an ill person by society, with exemption from normal social roles, and carrying specific rights and responsibilities (i.e. it is an external, social phenomenon).

Incapacity is reduced capacity for and functioning at work. It is difficult to distinguish between 'capacity' and 'performance' where the latter also depends on motivation and effort.

Note: This is not a simple causal chain. These are different elements of the human predicament that underlies sickness and disability benefits. For the social security system, the difficulty lies in discrepancies between the elements. It should also be noted that, in UK social security law, terms such as 'impairment' and 'disablement' have precise legal meanings.

Impairment is the most objective measure of a person's health condition, and is largely a medical definition, but it does not provide much information about how an individual is affected. Disability, on the other hand, is not just about a person's condition, but focuses on how their activities and participation are affected.

The question of how to define the complex phenomenon of 'disability' is at the heart of assessment for benefits. Concepts and definitions of disability vary, depending on what is being considered, from what perspective and for what purpose. The core of all definitions is limitation or restriction of normal activities, but the question is what underpins that limitation.

Earlier definitions of disability were based on a medical model, in which disability was regarded as a (more or less) direct consequence of an underlying impairment. Against this, commentators have argued that the medical model provides an inadequate basis for understanding the complex phenomenon of disability. In the context of disability rights, they have focused instead on the need for social change, and have proposed an alternative 'social model of disability', which essentially argues that many of the restrictions suffered by disabled people do not lie in their impairment, but are imposed by the way that society is organised for able-bodied living. This produces a very different definition of disability as:

 › *disadvantage* experienced by an individual . . .
 › . . . resulting from *barriers* to independent living or educational, employment or other opportunities . . .
 › . . . that impact on people with *impairments* and/or ill health.

This social focus may be most appropriate and useful for addressing disability rights, but it provides an insufficient basis for conceptualising individual entitlement to social security benefits. The current International Classification of Functioning, Disability and Health proposed by the World Health Organization recognises that the experience of disability is unique to the individual.

STATE BENEFITS

There is difficulty in defining 'incapacity for work' in the clinical context. Entitlement to benefits requires a cut-off point, but in reality there is a continuum with no sharp boundary between capacity and incapacity. Conditions and capacities change over time. There is a conceptual difference between those who 'can't carry out work activities' and those who 'can't get a job' in their relevant labour market because of their physical or mental condition. In practice there may be much overlap between the two. Personal factors, the social context and the impact of the social security system itself on human behaviour (including the moral hazard that 'financial benefits create dependency') may be excluded from the legal and administrative definition, but their importance cannot be denied.

The practical limitation of assessment is that it ultimately provides information about performance. It can never be an objective measure of what the claimant is *able* to do or *should be able* to do. As an over-simplification, capacity may be limited by physiology, but performance is limited by psychology – what the claimant does or does not do will always depend on effort and motivation.

Fitness for work advice, incapacity and certification

In the UK, for the first 7 days of illness or incapacity individuals certify their own unfitness for work using form SC1 (if they are unemployed or self-employed) or form SC2 (if they are employed). After the 7-day period, an official medical statement can be used by a registered medical practitioner to record the advice given to the patient in relation to their fitness for their regular occupation. Such statements are usually accepted as medical evidence by employers (who pay Statutory Sick Pay or the employer's equivalent) and by the Department for Work and Pensions (DWP), which administers state incapacity benefits.

Medical statements are official documents, and it is very important that they are completed in accordance with official guidance issued to all doctors by the DWP. Registered medical practitioners can issue the official statements (such as Med 3), but a wide range of other health professionals also provide advice on fitness to work for their patients. NHS general practitioners are required under their NHS Terms of Service to issue (or refuse to issue) statements to patients as an integral part of their clinical management of working-age patients. NHS GPs are also required to provide factual information about a patient who subsequently claims a state incapacity benefit to a DWP medical officer.

Form Med 3 is a statement of incapacity for work based on a medical examination of the patient on the day, or the day before, the certificate is issued. Within the first 6 months of incapacity the certificate can only be given for a period of up to 6 months or less. Certificates that are issued after the first 6 months can be given for longer periods. Provision is made on the Med 3 form for specification of a date for return to work, provided that it does not exceed 14 days from the day after the certificate is issued. A certificate which provides a period of incapacity but does not bear a return-to-work date is known as an 'open' certificate.

Where the patient is claiming a state incapacity benefit rather than Statutory Sick Pay (*see* page 153), the certifying doctor may be required to provide the patient with Form Med 4 on the first occasion that an independent medical assessment is applied. The information provided by the doctor on this form supplements that provided by the patient about how their health condition or disability impacts on their everyday life. It also provides an opportunity for the doctor to review the incapacity and, where appropriate, to advise a return to work.

The DWP Chief Medical Adviser issues guidance to all doctors which makes it clear that they should always consider carefully whether advising a patient to refrain from work is the most appropriate clinical management. Doctors may often best help a patient of working age by taking action that will encourage and support work retention and rehabilitation. The DWP guidance recommends that, when advising a patient about their fitness for work, doctors should consider the following factors:

> the nature of the patient's medical condition and how long it is expected to last
> the functional limitations which result from the patient's condition, particularly in relation to the types of tasks that they perform at work
> any reasonable adjustments which might enable the patient to continue working, noting that under the Disability Discrimination Act 1995 an employer may be required to make reasonable adjustments to the workplace for an employee with a long-term disability
> any appropriate clinical guidelines (e.g. the Royal College of General Practitioners has produced clinical guidelines on the management of acute low back pain, which emphasise the importance of remaining active)
> clinical management of the condition which is in the patient's best interest with regard to work fitness, including managing the patient's expectations in relation to their ability to continue working.

Form Med 3 may also be used to record advice that a patient need not refrain from work. For example, a doctor may use the 'Doctor's remarks' section to record that certain workplace adjustments may be appropriate or desirable in the light of the patient's medical condition or disability. If the GP thinks that further occupational health advice may be helpful, but does not feel confident to give it, he or she can suggest to the employer on the Med 3 form that advice from an occupational health practitioner would be advisable.

Full details on the medical evidence for Statutory Sick Pay, Statutory Maternity Pay and Social Security Incapacity Benefit can be found in *IB204: A Guide for Registered Medical Practitioners, 2004* (available at www.dwp.gov. uk/medical).

THE MAIN BENEFITS IN THE UK FOR PEOPLE WHO ARE UNABLE TO WORK DUE TO SICKNESS, INJURY OR DISABILITY

Statutory Sick Pay (SSP)

When absent from work because of illness, most employees receive either Statutory Sick Pay (SSP) or their employer's sick pay, which has to be an equivalent or better benefit. SSP is not a state benefit, but rather it is an obligation on employers overseen by the Inland Revenue. Those without an employer, namely the self-employed, unemployed and non-employed, and a few categories of employees who are not eligible for SSP, may claim a state incapacity benefit instead. SSP can be paid up to a maximum of 28 weeks. Spells of incapacity that are separated by a period of 8 weeks or less count as one. If the person is still incapable of work after SSP has been paid for 28 weeks, the person may transfer on to Incapacity Benefit. Shortly before the SSP is due to run out, an employer will give their employee a form with details of SSP paid. The form should be sent with a completed form SC1 to the benefit customer's, Jobcentre Plus or social security office.

Before paying SSP, an employer must be satisfied that the employee is incapable, because of a specific disease or disablement, of doing work that can reasonably be expected to be done under their contract of employment. In order to be paid a state incapacity benefit, the benefit customer must be suffering from a physical or mental disease or disablement. Therefore unless medical statements such as Form Med 3 indicate such a condition, the employer or the DWP may not be able to pay a benefit. Employees in receipt of SSP may apply to the Inland Revenue for National Insurance Credits for the period during which they are in receipt of payments. These credits protect their future benefit entitlement.

State incapacity benefits

The UK state incapacity benefits consist of a family of financial products, of which the main one is Incapacity Benefit itself. They are administered by an agency of the Department for Work and Pensions, Jobcentre Plus. In the UK in 2006, approximately 2.7 million adults of working age were on an Incapacity Benefit, representing 5% of the working-age population and a direct cost to taxpayers of £13 billion.

When a claim for a state incapacity benefit is made, there will at some point be a referral by Jobcentre Plus officials for independent medical advice. There are two tests of medical incapacity for work, defined in legislation, which are used for assessing entitlement to these benefits.

Own Occupation Test (OOT)

This test is only applicable for the first 28 weeks of incapacity, and only if the person has been engaged in paid work for at least 8 out of the last 21 weeks before the onset of incapacity. The test is designed to determine whether the person, by reason of some specific disease or bodily or mental disablement, is incapable of work which that person could reasonably be expected to do in the course of their occupation. Initially the OOT is satisfied by a valid medical statement, such as Med 3. Subsequently, an independent medical opinion on the person's fitness for their usual job will be sought.

The Personal Capability Assessment (PCA)

This test is applicable from the outset of incapacity if the Own Occupation Test does not apply (because the person has an insufficient record of recent work). For people who are subject to the OOT, the PCA will only apply after the benefit customer has been incapable of working for 28 weeks. For other individuals the PCA is applied from the start of their claim for an incapacity benefit. The PCA assesses the extent to which a person, by reason of some specific disease or bodily or mental disablement, is incapable of performing certain specified everyday activities (such as walking, standing, reaching, hearing and mental functions) set out in legislation. The level at which the threshold for benefit entitlement has been set has been designed to reflect the point at which a person's ability to perform work-related activities is substantially reduced, rather than the point at which work becomes impossible (*IB204: A Guide for Registered Medical Practitioners, 2004*; *IB214*).

Some people are treated as incapable of working without having to satisfy the OOT or PCA – for example, people who are exempt from the PCA on the grounds of very severe illness or disability, such as psychoses or terminal illness.

Incapacity Benefit

Entitlement for Incapacity Benefit is based on a person's National Insurance contributions, and is paid when a medical condition or disability prevents them from working. Benefit is paid at three different rates according to length of the spell of incapacity. The benefit is not 'means tested', but the two higher rates (normally paid after 28/52 weeks of incapacity) are taxable, and income from a pension over £85 per week is taken into account.

Income Support and Disability Premium payable to a person who is unable to work because of incapacity

This is a means-tested benefit, but it can be paid to those whose lack of National Insurance contributions prevents them from receiving Incapacity Benefit. Medical evidence such as Med 3 and the PCA may be used to support such claims.

National Insurance credits

People who are incapable of working but who are unable to claim other incapacity benefits can be credited with National Insurance, which helps to protect future entitlement to benefits such as state retirement pension. Again a Med 3 and PCA may be used as evidence in the assessment of entitlement.

Benefit Entitlement Decisions

Decisions on entitlement to statutory benefits are made by non-medical Decision Makers acting on behalf of the Secretary of State for Work and Pensions. Up until the time when the relevant test of incapacity (the OOT or the PCA) is applied, the Decision Maker will use the claimant's own doctor's statement (sick note) as medical evidence of incapacity for work.

Patients who meet the threshold of incapacity in the OOT or PCA

If the Decision-Maker determines that the claimant meets the threshold of incapacity, the certifying doctor will be informed of this by the Jobcentre Plus Office. In such circumstances the certifying doctor is no longer required to issue any statements to that patient in relation to the current claim to state incapacity benefit.

Patients who do not meet the threshold of incapacity under the OOT or PCA

If the claimant does not meet the threshold of incapacity (under the OOT or the PCA) they will not be able to receive a state incapacity benefit. The certifying doctor is no longer required to issue Med 3 statements except in certain defined circumstances, namely:

> if the patient's condition has deteriorated since the relevant assessment by the DWP

> if the diagnosed condition that is causing incapacity for work has changed significantly.

DISPUTES

A claimant can ask the DWP for an explanation of any benefit entitlement decision. If the claimant disagrees with the decision, they can ask the DWP for it to be reconsidered. Following a reconsideration, where the claimant continues to dispute the decision, they can have an appeal considered by an Appeal Tribunal, whose members are independent of the DWP. There may be a further right of appeal, if there is a question of an error of law, to a Social Security Commissioner.

Help to return to work

Jobcentre Plus provides access to a range of employment assessment and rehabilitative services specifically aimed at people on state incapacity benefits. Some examples are listed in Box 9.4. Clinicians can do much to encourage their patients to access and make use of these free services as part of their rehabilitative and recovery plan.

BOX 9.4 EXAMPLES OF EMPLOYMENT ASSESSMENT AND REHABILITATIVE SERVICES AVAILABLE THROUGH JOBCENTRE PLUS*

Disability Employment Advisers (DEAs) and other employment-focused Personal Advisers support people who, because of employment barriers associated with their disability, need specialist help. DEAs also work with employers in developing and implementing good employment practices with regard to recruiting and retaining disabled people.

Occupational psychologists provide tailored, employment-focused assessment for people who face barriers to work as a result of their disability or medical condition.

Permitted Work Rules allow people in receipt of a state incapacity benefit to do some work which may be therapeutic to their condition. Time and earnings limits apply, but permitted work may provide a valuable stepping stone from 'benefits' to mainstream work.

New Deal for Disabled People supports people in receipt of an incapacity or disability benefit in finding and retaining paid employment. It is a voluntary programme delivered through a network of Job Brokers from the public, private and voluntary sectors across England, Scotland and Wales.

Work Preparation is a scheme for those disabled people who are not yet ready to work, and who need help to build their skills and confidence in order to make effective occupational choices. For some, work preparation may include vocational training.

Access to Work aims to provide tailored support to individuals to help them to overcome the effects of disability at work (e.g. help with getting to work, making appropriate workplace adjustments, and the cost of aids and adaptations).

Job Introduction Scheme provides employers with a weekly grant towards the cost of employing people with disabilities for a trial period of employment of up to 13 weeks.

Workstep is the Government's supported employment programme, which aims to provide tailored support in finding, securing and retaining jobs for people with disabilities which give rise to more complex barriers to work. Workstep provides support and an opportunity for people to progress to open employment where this is appropriate for them.

* (www.jobcentreplus.gov.uk)

Working Tax Credit

The Working Tax Credit provides support to workers, including those who have a disability. The tax credits are payable for each eligible worker with a disability, thus improving work incentives. To be eligible, a person needs to work for at least 16 hours a week and to have a disability which puts them at a disadvantage in getting a job. There is a disability test, and the person must also have been in receipt of an incapacity benefit within the preceding 6 months (or be receiving Disability Living Allowance), their disability must be likely to last for 6 months, and their gross earnings must be 20% less than they were before the disability began. Further details are available from employers or from the Inland Revenue (www.inlandrevenue.gov.uk).

Jobseeker's Allowance (JSA)

Jobseeker's Allowance (JSA) is a benefit for people who are unemployed or who work for less than 16 hours a week and are looking for full-time work. It is not paid to people who are in full-time work (more than 16 hours a week), who may be able to claim a working tax credit. People with an illness, injury or disability who do not satisfy the appropriate test of incapacity for work may claim JSA, and it is possible to claim JSA and impose restrictions on the type of work or hours you are prepared to work because of your medical condition or disability. Unlike state incapacity benefits, JSA is time-limited.

Other state disability benefits for people of working age

Industrial Injuries Disablement Benefit

The main industrial injuries benefit is Industrial Injuries Disablement Benefit (IIDB), which is a form of 'no-fault' compensation provided by the State. To be eligible for an award under the state industrial injuries benefit scheme, a claimant must satisfy the *industrial injury condition* – that is:

› they were an employed earner
› they have suffered a personal injury in an industrial accident *or* they are suffering from a prescribed industrial disease, *and*
› as a result of that accident or disease they have suffered a *loss of faculty* (impairment of the proper functioning of part of the body or mind), *and*
› as a result of that loss of faculty they are disabled.

Discrete industrial accidents (e.g. back injury due to falling from a ladder) are covered, but injury by process (e.g. back injury due to misuse over a number of years) is not.

Prescribed diseases (e.g. PDA12 – carpal tunnel syndrome) are recognised for particular occupations. The claimant must prove:

› that they have worked in one or more of the jobs for which that disease is prescribed (prescribed occupations), *and*
› that the job caused the disease.

A person qualifies for IIDB if:

› they satisfy the *industrial condition* as a result of one or more industrial accidents or prescribed diseases
› the resulting disablement is assessed as being at least 14% (1% in certain prescribed lung diseases, and 20% in occupational deafness), *and*
› 90 days have elapsed since the date of the accident or the onset of the prescribed disease.

There is no rehabilitative element in IIDB. It simply provides some financial compensation. If an individual is incapacitated for work, they may also claim a state incapacity benefit or Jobseeker's Allowance and access the full range of support services offered by Jobcentre Plus.

Disability Living Allowance

Disability Living Allowance (DLA) and Attendance Allowance (AA) are social security benefits intended to contribute to the extra costs resulting from a severe disability. Entitlement is based upon the help needed with personal care (e.g. washing, dressing, bathing, etc.), or the need for supervision or help with getting around. It does not include help with activities such as shopping or housework. The benefit is independent of income, National Insurance contributions or employment, so unlike the situation with state incapacity benefits, people *can be working* and still receive DLA. DLA is available to those who are under the age of 65 years, although if entitlement is established before that age, payment will continue after 65 years. AA is available to those over 65 years of age. DLA has no rehabilitative component – it simply provides money. Those who have an incapacity for work may also claim a state incapacity benefit and be eligible for the job preparation and job search support available to such claimants through Jobcentre Plus.

DLA has two components:

❯ **mobility** – paid at two rates:
- higher – for those who are unable to walk or virtually unable to walk
- lower – for those who are unable to find their way around in unfamiliar places without guidance or supervision (those people with a mental health or sensory impairment)

❯ **care** – paid at three rates:
- lower – for those who need attention or supervision for a significant proportion of the day, or who are unable to plan and prepare a cooked main meal
- middle – for those who need frequent attention or supervision throughout the day, or repeated and prolonged attention throughout the night, or who need to be watched over at night
- higher – for those who need help throughout both day and night.

Decisions about benefit entitlement are made by non-medical DWP staff called Decision Makers (DMs). The role of the DM is to consider all of the available evidence and make a decision on benefit entitlement in accordance with the relevant legislation.

CONCLUSION

The UK state benefit system is continually being reformed in order to better meet the needs of individuals who face barriers to work because of illness, injury or disability. The assessment of incapacity and support needs is complex, and depends on disability, capacity and performance rather than simply the underlying impairment. Medical assessments based within a tight legal framework are used to assess entitlement to state benefits so as to ensure fairness and equity of access. Work is an important part of everyday life, and can bring benefits to individuals, their families and wider society. Work rehabilitative services are increasingly open to a wider group of disabled people who have the capacity and the desire to work.

REFERENCES

1 Waddell G, Aylward M. *The Scientific and Conceptual Basis of Incapacity Benefits.* London: The Stationery Office; 2005.
2 Waddell G, Burton AK. *Concepts of Rehabilitation for the Management of Common Health Problems.* London: The Stationery Office; 2004.

FURTHER READING

The Department for Work and Pensions website (www.dwp.gov.uk/medical) is an excellent source of information for healthcare professionals advising on capacity for work in the UK. It provides information on statutory certification and the relevant benefits and assessment procedures. This is *essential* information both for NHS general practitioners and for occupational health professionals. The site also provides online training, guidance notes and a section on 'Frequently asked questions.'
IB204: a guide for registered medical practitioners; www.dwp.gov.uk/medical/guides (accessed March 2008)
Waddell G, Burton AK. *Concepts of Rehabilitation for the Management of Common Health Problems.* London: The Stationery Office; 2004.
Waddell G, Aylward M. *The Scientific and Conceptual Basis of Incapacity Benefits.* London: The Stationery Office; 2005.

CHAPTER 10

The legal framework

The function of legal rules and procedures in the field of health and safety at work and disability is to deter by punishing infringements of the criminal law, and to provide compensation through the civil law system for the victims of unlawful treatment. In addition, entitlement to welfare benefits is conferred on those who are unable to work due to sickness or injury. Rehabilitation plays little part in any of these scenarios. Indeed, as has been commented elsewhere in this book, the pursuit of compensation may be a deterrent to a return to work, since the level of compensation depends on the degree of disability. Those engaged in legal proceedings will be unable to put the past behind them until the proceedings are over, and this will take many months, if not years. Furthermore, an award of compensation can be a mixed blessing, since it may remove one of the incentives to return to employment which, in the long run, is not for the benefit of the individual, who loses the society of work colleagues and the social status of being economically productive – a giver rather than a taker.

In this chapter an attempt will be made to set out the legal framework in order to highlight to readers, mainly employers and health professionals, how legal duties impact on their responsibilities to employees and patients.

THE DUTY OF CARE OF A HEALTH PROFESSIONAL

Doctors and nurses are subject to the criminal law in the same way as other members of society. If they are employers, they have the same obligations to comply with health and safety legislation as any other employer, and are subject to enforcement proceedings through the criminal courts. Gross negligence which causes a death may lead to a conviction in a criminal court for the crime of manslaughter.

All health professionals owe a duty of care at common law (the law made by the courts through precedent rather than by Parliament) to their patients. This is civil law, for which the remedy is the payment of money damages. The duty is to take reasonable care to prevent foreseeable damage. The question of what a reasonable doctor or nurse should have done is determined by the standards of the profession.[1] Expert witnesses will be asked to advise on what was reasonable in the circumstances of the case. An error is not necessarily proof of negligence, if in the circumstances it was a reasonable thing to do.

In addition to this legal duty, the professions themselves have created ethical standards by which members of the professions will be judged. The sanction for a serious failure to comply with professional standards is removal from the professional register. Professional bodies have created disciplinary procedures to adjudicate on allegations of misconduct. Their decisions can be appealed to the High Court. The Council for Regulatory Excellence,[2] set up under the NHS Reform and Healthcare Professions Act 2002, has power to refer to the High Court a decision of a professional body that is thought to be too lenient. At the time of writing, the disciplinary role of the professional bodies remains under review.

The duty of care is primarily to prevent physical damage. The courts are less willing to hold that there is a duty to prevent economic loss. This is especially important where the doctor's or nurse's report will lead to refusal or loss of a job. In *Kapfunde v Abbey National*,[3] a part-time occupational physician who had no clinical relationship with job applicants reported to an employer that Mrs Kapfunde, who was applying for a job, would be likely to have a higher than average sickness absence level. She had stated on her pre-employment questionnaire that she suffered from sickle-cell anaemia, and had had several weeks of sickness absence in the previous two years. Mrs Kapfunde sued the doctor for negligence when she was not appointed to the job. The Court of Appeal held that the doctor was not negligent because her advice was reasonable, but that in any event she owed no duty of care to a job applicant to prevent economic loss. Her duty was to the employer alone. (This case arose before the Disability Discrimination Act 1995 came into force. There might now be a claim under that Act.)

It is likely that the courts would hold that a general practitioner who completes a Form Med 3 does not owe a duty of care to the patient, since it is for the purpose only of claiming Statutory Sick Pay, but this does not apply to a medical report sent to the employer on which the employer relies when making employment decisions. The existence of a clinical relationship probably imparts a duty to exercise reasonable care when writing such reports (e.g. by providing accurate information).

Employers are in general not liable in criminal law for the acts of their employees, but they are vicariously liable for the civil wrongdoing of those directly employed, if it occurred in the course of employment. A GP is vicariously liable for the negligence of a practice nurse, as well as that of his partners, but not for the negligence of a deputising doctor.

DUTIES OF THE EMPLOYER

All those who employ staff directly are subject to these laws, including general practitioners and NHS trusts. There are also legal duties towards those who are not directly employed, but who may be affected by the employer's activities – for example, the employees of contractors and members of the public visiting the employer's premises.

These can be divided into:

> Duties imposed by statute, both primary legislation, such as the Health and Safety at Work Act 1974 (HSWA), and secondary legislation in the form of statutory instruments, such as the Control of Substances Hazardous to Health Regulations 2002 (COSHH). Regulations are the detailed provisions which Parliament uses to put flesh on the bare bones of the parent Act.
> Duties imposed by the common law, i.e. judge-made law created in case law, not imposed by statute or statutory instrument.

Health and safety statutes and regulations impose criminal liability. The employer is subject to enforcement procedures invoked by public officials from the Health and Safety Executive and local authorities. The ultimate sanction is prosecution in a criminal court (either the magistrates' court or the Crown Court in England and Wales). Conviction leads in most cases to punishment by the imposition of a fine, although imprisonment of a manager is also a possibility.

The common law, on the other hand, is concerned mainly with compensation. The tort (delict in Scotland) of negligence imposes a common law duty on the employer to take reasonable care of employees and others within the foreseeable area of risk, like employees of contractors. Enforcement of this duty is not a matter for public officials. The claimant who has been injured by a failure of care must sue for damages in the civil courts (either the County

Court or the High Court). In many cases, damages are paid by an insurance company. The civil action should be contrasted with entitlement to Industrial Injuries Disablement Benefit, where the claimant does not have to show that the employer was at fault. A claimant who is successful in the tort action and is awarded damages must reimburse the Department for Work and Pensions for the social security benefits received over 5 years.[4]

In addition to the tort of negligence, there is the tort of breach of statutory duty. Where the employer is in breach of some statutes or statutory regulations, the injured claimant can sue in a civil court for damages for that breach, in addition to or instead of a possible criminal prosecution brought in the criminal court. Not all statutes give rise to an action for breach of statutory duty. In the field of health and safety at work, the Health and Safety at Work Act 1974 (HSWA) itself does not afford such an action, but most of the statutory regulations (e.g. COSHH, Manual Handling, Noise at Work) do.

CRIMINAL LIABILITY

Virtually all criminal law is in the form of statute. The principal health and safety legislation is the HSWA. Since 1974 the Act has been supplemented by a number of different regulations relating to specific hazards, many of which stem from European Community directives. In European Community law, a qualified majority of Member States voting in the Council of Ministers can impose minimum health and safety obligations throughout the European Union against the wishes of the minority. This is in order to create a level playing field for commerce and industry throughout the common market. Member States are under a legal obligation to introduce domestic legislation implementing European directives passed by the Council.

The most important regulations are the Management of Health and Safety at Work Regulations, originally passed in 1992, but updated in 1999. These implement the European Framework Directive.

Separate from the health and safety legislation is the general criminal law, including the common-law crime of manslaughter – that is, the killing of a human being by reckless conduct or gross negligence. For an employer to be convicted of this crime it had to be proved that a very senior manager (one who decides policy) was at fault. This proved difficult in cases involving large organisations where responsibility is shared, such as train-operating companies. As a result, a new crime of corporate killing has been created, consisting of a management failure by a corporation which falls far below what can reasonably be expected and which causes someone's death. In

2007, the Corporate Manslaughter and Corporate Homicide Act became law, implementing these changes.

From April 2008, a company, but not an individual, can be prosecuted and fined for this new crime, in addition to offences under the Health and Safety at Work Act. It remains possible for an individual to be prosecuted and convicted for common law manslaughter, and there have been several prosecutions of doctors and nurses for that offence.

The aim of criminal sanctions is to deter and to punish wrongdoing, not to provide a route to compensation. That is the function of the civil law.

HEALTH AND SAFETY COMMISSION AND HEALTH AND SAFETY EXECUTIVE

The Health and Safety Commission (HSC) is a part-time body consisting of employer and employee representatives and independent members. It is the main health and safety policy-making body in the UK, and is responsible for helping to draft new legislation and approving Codes of Practice. The Health and Safety Executive (HSE) is responsible to the HSC for enforcement of the safety laws. In addition, the local authority environmental health officers police offices, shops, hotels and catering establishments. Both of these bodies came under the general supervision of the Department for Work and Pensions in 2002. It is proposed to combine the HSC and the HSE.

The HSE and local authority inspectors have the power to inspect premises and issue improvement and prohibition notices. An improvement notice orders the recipient to take remedial steps (e.g. to guard a machine) within a specified period. A prohibition notice orders the discontinuance of an activity where it involves a risk of serious personal injury. It can be imposed with immediate effect. Prosecutions are reserved for offences of a flagrant, wilful or reckless nature. Magistrates can impose fines of up to £20 000, but the Crown Court (or the High Court in Scotland) can impose an unlimited fine. In 2005, a Scottish judge ordered Transco to pay £15 million for its part in a gas explosion that killed a family of four.

DUTIES UNDER THE CRIMINAL LAW

The employer must ensure, so far as is reasonably practicable, the health, safety and welfare at work of its employees (Section 2 of the HSWA). Health includes both physical and mental health. In addition, employers must do what is reasonably practicable to protect individuals who are not employed by them, such as sub-contractors and members of the public, who may be affected by their activities (Section 3 of the HSWA). Reasonable practicability involves a cost-benefit analysis. The greater the risk, the more resources must be expended to protect those at risk.

A professional whose incompetent advice leads to the employer breaching health and safety laws can be prosecuted either instead of, or as well as, the employer. One example was the conviction of an occupational hygienist whose incompetence led to the unlawful exposure of employees in a factory to high levels of wood dust. An occupational health specialist acting as a consultant runs the risk of a similar prosecution. Employees also have a duty to take reasonable care for their own health and safety and that of other individuals who may be affected by their acts or omissions at work (Section 7 of the HSWA).

Statutory regulations make more detailed provision for specific activities and hazards. They are often accompanied by an Approved Code of Practice (ACOP) giving detailed guidance approved by the Health and Safety Commission. The HSWA provides that breach of an ACOP is evidence of a breach of the law, unless the defendant can prove that he used equally effective means to promote safety.

Guidance from the HSE does not have the same authority as an ACOP, but nevertheless will be taken into account if a case reaches a court of law. For example, in 2004 the HSE developed standards against which management can measure its performance in protecting workers against stress-related illness.[5] The Management of Health and Safety at Work Regulations and ACOP 1999 lay down the following broad general principles for the management of health and safety.

> Every employer shall make a suitable and sufficient risk assessment.
> Where there are five or more employees, records must be kept.
> Consideration must be given to workers especially at risk, including pregnant workers, young workers, and workers with a disability.
> Every employer shall ensure that his employees are provided with such health surveillance as is appropriate, having regard to the risks to their health and safety identified by the risk assessment.
> Where workers are returning to work on a programme of gradual rehabilitation, special consideration will have to be given to their needs.

LAW OF COMPENSATION: CIVIL LIABILITY

The civil law of tort or delict is concerned with compensation. The aim is to make up to the injured person with a money payment the loss he has incurred, in so far as that is possible. Until very recently, payment has been in the form of a lump sum of damages, and the issue of rehabilitation has played no part. There have been sad cases where compensation has run out before the injured person's death, and where the injured person has been exploited by unscrupulous individuals in pursuit of his or her capital sum. On the other hand, there have been cases where the claimant unexpectedly died shortly after having received a large award, which then passed to his surviving relatives.

Since 1990 an award of damages can be made by way of a structured settlement whereby the bulk of the money is paid through an annuity. The Inland Revenue has agreed to treat the annuity payments as tax-exempt payments of capital. In the Courts Act 2003 there is now a general power to award periodical payments instead of a lump sum of damages for personal injury, but the court may only do this where the continuity of payments is reasonably guaranteed. It is presumed that a government or health service body is reliable for this purpose.

By the Employers' Liability (Compulsory Insurance) Act 1969, most employers are compelled by law to insure against actions by their employees for work-related injury, and there is a criminal penalty for failure to comply. A comprehensive review of employers' liability insurance has been undertaken by the Department for Work and Pensions, and two reports were published (in 2003 and 2004). These point out that in other countries (e.g. Germany) the insurance company first pays for medical intervention intended to return the injured party to reasonable health. Only when the outcome of this intervention has been seen is the final level of compensation for the degree of disability assessed. A further difficulty is that employers' liability insurance covers the employer only where there is legal liability – that is, in most cases where there is negligence. Yet rehabilitation needs to commence as soon as possible, probably before liability has been established. Who is to pay for treatment in cases where there is no proof that the employer was at fault?

Much of the cost of insurance cover is taken up by legal fees. The prohibitive costs of pursuing an action in the civil courts have been reduced by reforms to civil procedure recommended by a committee chaired by Lord Woolf, a senior judge. The new Civil Procedure Rules came into effect in 1999. These rules place greater emphasis on pre-action negotiation to encourage an agreed settlement. Parties who refuse to negotiate may be penalised in costs. The judge has increased powers of case management to try to keep the proceedings on the move. In most cases of negligence a single expert witness will be instructed, rather than each party using separate experts. There is a fast-track system for personal injury claims up to a value of £15 000. There has been an increase in the number of claims which the parties agree to submit to Alternative Dispute Resolution, usually engaging the services of a mediator who will try to suggest a compromise to which both parties can agree.

The common law of negligence imposes a duty on the employer to take reasonable care to prevent foreseeable damage. This is threefold – to provide safe plant and equipment, safe personnel and a safe system of work. What is reasonable depends on the facts of each case, and risk must be balanced against the cost of avoiding it. In recent years there has been a sharp increase in the number of claims for work-related ill health, including deafness, hand–arm vibration syndrome, work-related upper limb disorders and work-related stress. In *Sutherland v Hatton*[6] the Court of Appeal laid down guidelines for the courts dealing with mental health cases, and these were subsequently approved by the House of Lords in *Barber v Somerset County Council*.[7] It was emphasised that the employee must prove that the employer should have foreseen the possibility of ill health caused by work. If the employee has kept his symptoms secret from the employer, it will be difficult to establish this fore-seeability. In *Hartman v South Essex Community Care and Mental Health NHS Trust*,[8] the Court of Appeal held that, where a care assistant had confided her history of depressive illness to her employer's occupational health adviser, the employer was not deemed to have knowledge of her vulnerability because the occupational health department had a strict duty of confidentiality in relation to clinical information.

There are no 'Stress Regulations', but many other occupational diseases are covered by statutory regulations and/or Approved Codes of Practice. Where there are regulations, the injured employee can sue for breach of statutory duty as well as for common-law negligence. The wording of the regulations may be held to import strict liability – that is, it will be unnecessary to prove negligence. In *Dugmore v Swansea NHS Trust*,[9] a theatre nurse developed an allergy to latex protein while using powdered latex gloves in the course of her work. At the time, this hazard was not generally appreciated. The court held that the employer was not negligent, but decided that it was liable for breach of the COSHH Regulations, which imposed no-fault liability. Regulation 7(1) provides that 'Every employer shall ensure that the exposure of his employees to a substance hazardous to health is either prevented or, where this is not reasonably practicable, adequately controlled.' Control had been inadequate, so the employer was liable.

LAW OF COMPENSATION: WELFARE BENEFITS

State benefits for those who are unable to work due to an industrial injury are of two kinds, namely regular payments to support the worker during absence from work, and a disablement pension to compensate for permanent disability. Much of this has already been covered in Chapter 9. The main differences between the State scheme and the civil tort action are as follows:

❭ the State scheme is funded through taxation, whereas the tort action is mostly funded by private insurance companies

❭ the State scheme is a no-fault scheme – that is, payments are due whether or not the employer was at fault in causing the worker's injury

❭ the State scheme gives regular payments which can be varied if the worker's condition improves or deteriorates

❭ the State scheme has its own adjudication procedures, separate from the civil courts.

EMPLOYMENT LAW

Most of employment law is the creature of statute and has come into being in the last 40 years. It has its own separate court system – the employment tribunals. The tribunals' jurisdiction is principally unfair dismissal (Employment Rights Act 1996) and the anti-discrimination statutes, prohibiting discrimination on grounds of sex, marital status, race, disability, religion, sexual orientation or age. Much of employment law originates in European Community directives, so that the ultimate court of appeal is the European Court of Justice in Luxembourg. The statutory provisions are supplemented by Codes of Practice which are not themselves the law, but which may be taken into account by courts and tribunals in deciding cases. These are often drafted by the Advisory, Conciliation and Arbitration Service (ACAS). Other important bodies in the past were the Equal Opportunities Commission (sex discrimination), the Commission for Racial Equality (race discrimination) and the Disability Rights Commission (disability discrimination). In 2007 these were merged into a Commission for Equality and Human Rights. Northern Ireland has its own Equality Commission.

SICK PAY

The employer has a duty to pay Statutory Sick Pay (SSP) to employees for up to 28 weeks. No statutory payment is due for the first 3 days of absence. The administration of SSP is under the control of the Inland Revenue. In addition to SSP, the contract of employment may oblige the employer to make up SSP to full wages for at least a period, but this is not obligatory. In the public sector it is common for the contract to entitle the employee to full pay for 6 months and half pay for a further 6 months. In the private sector, employees who are entitled to more than SSP are fortunate.

The courts have held that where an employee is covered by a permanent health insurance scheme, there is an implied term in the contract that the employer will not dismiss him while he is off sick. This does not prevent the employer from dismissing for misconduct or redundancy. In *Briscoe v Lubrizol Ltd*,[10] the employee was absent for a long period. The scheme was financed through an insurance company. In 1991 the insurance company refused to continue paying on the ground that Briscoe was not medically unfit. The employer sent him to its occupational health physician, who referred him to a specialist. The specialist's report did not support Briscoe's assertion that he was unfit for his normal occupation. The employee continued to be absent from work, supported by his GP, and refused to meet his managers or answer their phone calls. He was dismissed for misconduct in not replying to his employer's reasonable requests and instructions. This was held to be a fair dismissal, which effectively terminated any right that Briscoe had to insurance benefits.

Employers are not entitled to ask for a doctor's certificate for the first 7 days of absence, but after that general practitioners are at present obliged to certify sickness absence on the Med 3 form. Proposals to remove this responsibility are discussed elsewhere in this book. Many employers use a system of self-certification for an absence of less than 7 days.

Although the statutory certificate is issued for the purpose of access to State benefits, it is widely regarded – and this includes employment tribunals – as evidence that the employee's illness is genuine. Where it can be proved that the employee is malingering there is, of course, no right to sick pay, and the employer can discipline the employee for gross misconduct. Employers are advised not to accuse an employee of lying unless they have evidence that this is the case. Occasionally, there is a disagreement between the GP and the employer's occupational health physician. In *Scottish Courage Ltd v Guthrie*,[11] Guthrie was a driver/drayman who had had an accident at work and was signed off by his GP for 4 weeks. The company medical adviser who saw him said that he was fit for work from 27 February, but the GP gave him another medical certificate up until 10 March. The employer refused to pay contractual sick pay for the last 5 days of absence. The contract of employment stated that employees were entitled to full pay if absent due to illness, but on condition that management was satisfied that the sickness was genuine. Neither doctor reported that the illness was not genuine. It was held on interpretation of the contract that the employee was entitled to sick pay for the last week of absence. However, if there had been evidence of malingering, the employer would not have been bound by the GP's certificate. The employer is in most cases entitled to prefer the report of its occupational health physician, who is more familiar with the demands of the job than is the GP. In a case of conflict, it may be advisable to send the employee to an independent specialist for a report, although this can be expensive and time-consuming.

Occasionally, a manager who is suspicious will resort to covert surveillance. The courts have held that this is not a breach of the Human Rights Act, and that evidence obtained by these means is admissible in court and tribunal proceedings.[12]

SICKNESS ABSENCE

Gone are the bad old days when an employee could be lawfully dismissed merely because he was off sick for a short time. However, as has been pointed out elsewhere in this book, it may not be in the employee's best interests in the long term to be left at home on sick pay without any contact with his manager or any attempt at rehabilitation.

After a lengthy period of sickness absence, the employer may come to the conclusion that they will have to dispense with the employee's services. This is not necessarily unfair. The employer has the right under the Employment Rights Act 1996 to dismiss an employee whose ill health makes him incapable of doing the job, so long as they follow a fair procedure. What is reasonable depends on the job, the length of service of the employee, the length of sickness absence and the medical prognosis. It is not true that an employee cannot be lawfully dismissed while he has a medical certificate from his GP. It is also not true that he cannot be dismissed while still receiving sick pay, although employers are normally expected to wait until sick pay is exhausted before making the decision to dismiss. To be fair, the employer must obtain medical evidence, consult with the employee or his representative and try to find an alternative job, if one is available. The leading case on dismissal for ill health is *East Lindsey District Council v Daubney*,[13] where a surveyor was dismissed after long periods of sickness absence due to anxiety and general debility. The personnel director had sought medical advice from the district community physician, who wrote that the employee was unfit to carry out his duties and should be retired on the ground of permanent ill health, and acted on it without indicating to the employee that his job might be at risk or allowing him to obtain his own doctor's report. The dismissal was held to be unfair.

An employee who complains to an employment tribunal that he or she has been unfairly dismissed must have worked for the employer continuously for at least a year at the date of dismissal. There is an upper limit on the compensatory award for unfair dismissal (£60 600 in 2007). Compensation cannot be given for injury to feelings, merely for financial loss. It is common for claimants to submit claims for both unfair dismissal and disability discrimination in the same proceedings, but they cannot obtain double damages.

Since the Disability Discrimination Act 1995 came into force, the employer of a person with a disability has a duty to make reasonable adjustments to the working environment or any provision, criterion or practice (see below).

Intermittent short-term absences for a series of ostensibly minor complaints such as colds and stomach upsets need different treatment. If the level of sickness absence is unacceptably high, the employer should first ask for a medical report in case there is an underlying chronic condition. If the response is negative, the employer should issue warnings that if attendance does not improve, dismissal is likely. In *Wilson v Post Office*,[14] the Court of Appeal held that dismissal for intermittent sickness absence after warnings is not for misconduct or incapability, but for 'some other substantial reason' under the Employment Rights Act 1996.

It is automatically unfair to refuse to employ, to dismiss or to discriminate against a woman because she may become or is pregnant, has given birth, has taken maternity leave or is breastfeeding. This is a form of sex discrimination and it cannot be justified, however inconvenient the employee's maternity leave may be to the employer, especially the small employer.

DISABILITY DISCRIMINATION ACT 1995

This is probably the most important legislation from the point of view of rehabilitation. Before it came into force, the only statutes protecting the disabled were the Disabled Persons (Employment) Acts 1944 and 1958, which obliged employers to employ a quota of registered disabled people. These statutes have been repealed. There is now no quota system and no register of the disabled for employment purposes.

The Disability Discrimination Act 1995 (Amendment) Regulations 2003 extended the Act to all employees except for the armed forces. It is no longer relevant that the employer employs only a few employees. The Act applies to the police, the fire service and the prison service. A disabled person is defined as a person with a physical or mental impairment which has a substantial and long-term adverse effect on his ability to carry out normal day-to-day activities. A substantial adverse effect is one which is more than minor or trivial. 'Long-term' means having lasted 12 months or more, likely to last 12 months or more, or terminal. Normal day-to-day activities are mobility, manual dexterity, physical coordination, continence, ability to lift, carry or otherwise move everyday objects, speech, hearing and eyesight, memory or ability to concentrate, learn or understand, and perception of the risk of physical danger. The Act is supplemented by Codes of Practice drafted by the Disability Rights Commission, the most important of which is the Code of Practice: Employment and Occupation, which was updated in 2004. The Code is not the law, but may be taken into account in courts and tribunals.

The Disability Discrimination Act 2005 removes the requirement for a mental impairment caused by mental illness to be a clinically well recognised illness. It also makes HIV infection, multiple sclerosis and cancer disabilities from the date of onset. Other progressive conditions count as disabilities from the time when symptoms become significant, even though they are not yet disabling. Where a condition such as diabetes or epilepsy is controlled by medication, the person is deemed to be disabled if he or she would be substantially impaired without the drugs. A disability which is assisted by a prosthesis (e.g. a hearing aid or artificial limb) is assessed without the artificial aid, apart from defects in eyesight, where spectacles or contact lenses are taken into account when assessing the degree of disability. Past disabilities count even though the person has now recovered from them (this is particularly important in the case of mental illness). Certain antisocial conditions, such as alcoholism, drug addiction, kleptomania and paedophilia, are not protected by the Act. Although medical evidence may be important in assessing the nature and degree of impairment, and its effect on the individual, the ultimate decision as to whether someone falls within the definition of disability in the Act is for the tribunal, not the doctor, who should therefore write a report in terms of a possible disability, rather than making a definite judgment.

Five kinds of discrimination are prohibited by the Act. The first is direct discrimination – that is, treating the person less favourably simply because of the fact of disability (e.g. excluding an applicant from becoming a police officer because they have insulin-dependent diabetes). Each person must be assessed individually. The second kind of discrimination is disability related – that is, treating the person less favourably because of one of the consequences of the disability (e.g. above average sickness absence or clumsiness). The third kind of discrimination is failure to make a reasonable adjustment to the working environment or a provision, criterion or practice to allow the disabled person to work. The fourth kind of discrimination is harassing a person with a disability (e.g. calling him unpleasant names), and the fifth kind is victimisation – that is, punishing a disabled person for complaining about the way they have been treated.

Disability-related discrimination can be justified by showing that the employer has a material and substantial reason, which may be that the effects of the disability make the disabled person an unacceptable health and safety risk. If the employer has undertaken a proper risk assessment performed by a competent person, that constitutes justification, as in *Jones v Post Office*,[15] where an insulin-dependent diabetic with a Class 1 licence was permitted to drive a small van for only 2 hours a day after a risk assessment performed by a Fellow of the Faculty of Occupational Medicine. The tribunal was not permitted to rely on medical evidence from a consultant who disagreed with the occupational physician to overturn the risk assessment. The tribunal does not have the general power to make its own appraisal of the medical evidence, or to conclude that the evidence from admittedly suitably competent medical advisers relied on by the employer was wrong, or to make its own risk assessment, even if the tribunal thinks that the employer's reason was based on inferior medical evidence.

Another possible justification may be proof that the disabled person's sickness absence is so protracted that it has become an unacceptable burden for the employer, but the employer is expected to tolerate more sickness absence caused by disability than normal levels of absence. Each case depends on its facts.

The other forms of discrimination cannot be justified.

The duty of reasonable adjustment is the issue most often raised before tribunals, and is the most relevant to rehabilitation. The employer must take any reasonable steps to remove the disabled person's disadvantage so that he or she can compete on a level footing. The Disability Discrimination Act requires positive discrimination, which is generally unlawful in other areas of discrimination, such as gender and race. A good example is *Archibald v Fife Council*,[16] where an employee road sweeper had impaired mobility after an operation went wrong. The Council trained her in basic secretarial skills, in which she was competent, but then insisted that she compete with other job applicants for low-grade secretarial posts which were a grade higher than her previous job. She applied for 100 jobs with the Council, but was not appointed. The House of Lords held that the employer should have considered appointing her to a vacant secretarial post without a competitive interview, giving her preference over other job applicants, as part of the duty of reasonable adjustment.

The duty is to make adjustments to both the physical environment and any provision, criterion or practice. The Act cites the following as examples of adjustments which may be considered:

- making alterations to premises
- allocating some of the disabled person's duties to another person
- transferring him to fill an existing vacancy
- altering hours of working and training
- assigning him to a different place of work or training
- allowing him to be absent during working or training hours for rehabilitation, assessment or treatment
- giving him, or arranging for, training or mentoring (whether for the disabled person or any other person)
- acquiring or modifying equipment
- modifying instructions or reference manuals
- modifying procedures for testing or assessment
- providing a reader or interpreter, or providing supervision or other support.

The duty is not absolute. In the first place it only applies where the employer either knows, or can reasonably be expected to know, that a job applicant or person in employment has a disability. Secondly, the employer only has to do that which is reasonable, taking into account the following factors:

- the extent to which taking the step would prevent the effect in question
- the extent to which it is practicable for the employer to take the step
- the financial and other costs which would be incurred by the employer in taking the step, and the extent to which taking it would disrupt any of his activities
- the extent of the employer's financial and other resources
- the availability to the employer of financial or other assistance with regard to taking the step
- the nature of his activities and the size of his undertaking
- where the step would be taken in relation to a private household, the extent to which taking it would:
  - disrupt the household, *or*
  - disturb any person residing there.

Employers are expected to research the availability of grants from the Access to Work fund which makes moneys available to support disabled workers or job applicants. In *Smith v Churchills Stairlifts plc*,[17] Smith was disabled with lumbar spondylosis which precluded him from lifting and carrying heavy objects. He applied for a job as a sales surveyor of radiator cabinets. He was turned down for the job because he would be unable to carry a full-sized demonstration radiator cabinet when visiting customers' premises. Smith asked whether he could use a miniature version on a trial basis, but this request was refused. It was held by the Court of Appeal that the employer had failed to make a reasonable adjustment and was liable for disability discrimination.

The employer is not obliged to create a job for an employee who has become disabled in employment. However, they are required to consider whether the worker could continue with his old job if reasonable adjustments were made. Perhaps a minor part of the employee's duties could be done by someone else, or he could work flexitime, or he could be provided with special equipment. If these options are not feasible, the employer should ask whether suitable alternative work could be made available. It may be necessary for the employee to be provided with training. The Code of Practice advises that the employer is entitled to ask whether the employee will remain in the job for long enough to justify the costs of training.

An important recent decision is *Meikle v Nottinghamshire County Council*.[18] A partially sighted schoolteacher asked for better lighting and large-print documents, and went off sick with stress when these were not provided. After a year she resigned. It was held that she was entitled to full pay for the year she was off sick, because it was the employer's failure to make a reasonable adjustment which had caused her absence. It remains to be seen how far this principle will be developed by the courts. Certainly employers are advised that they should not treat disability-related absence (e.g. for treatment or training) as sick leave, and that they should be willing to be more flexible about the amount of sickness absence of disabled workers than they are about that of the non-disabled.

However, if an employee is given unlimited sick pay when absent because of a disability-related illness, there will be little incentive to return to work. The Court of Appeal in *O'Hanlon v Commissioners for Inland Revenue and Customs*[19] considered the case of an employee who was disabled with chronic depression. She took 365 days off sick in 4 years, of which 320 days related to her disability and 45 days related to other medical conditions. She was paid 6 months full pay and 6 months half pay, but thereafter was on the pension rate of pay. She claimed that her employer had failed to make a reasonable adjustment to her pay, and that she should have received full pay for all disability-related sickness absences. She also submitted that all of her disability-related absences should be excluded from her record of days of sickness absence. The employer gave evidence that, were it to adopt the practices she was advocating for disabled employees, it would cost the Department around £6 million a year. The court held that the employer was not obliged to accede to the employee's requests as part of its duty of reasonable adjustment. As was stated in the Employment Appeal Tribunal:

> the purpose of this legislation is to assist the disabled to obtain employment and to integrate them into the workforce . . . The Act is designed to recognise the dignity of the disabled and to require modifications which will enable them to play a full part in the world of work, important and laudable aims. It is not to treat them as objects of charity which, as the tribunal pointed out, may in fact sometimes and for some people tend to act as a positive disincentive to return to work.

The employer must be flexible, but does not have to tolerate unlimited sickness absence because the worker has a disability. Much will depend on the type of job and the medical prognosis. In *Callagan v Glasgow City Council*,[20] a residential social worker was dismissed after 3 years' absence with a stress-related illness. The employer had tried to set up meetings with him to discuss the situation, but the employee refused to cooperate. The doctor was unable to give a date when he was likely to be able to return to work. It was held that his dismissal was justified.

The Code of Practice gives a number of examples of reasonable adjustments. These could include allowing a disabled person to work flexible hours to enable him to have additional breaks to overcome fatigue, permitting part-time working, a phased return to work with a gradual build-up of hours, allowing him to have additional time off for rehabilitation training, moving him to a different job, providing special equipment, providing a support worker, and so on. When someone has become disabled in employment, it may be that productivity will be impaired. The Code suggests that employers should be flexible with regard to payment arrangements. For example, a disabled person who is paid purely on the basis of output needs frequent short breaks. It is likely to be a reasonable adjustment for their employer to pay them at an agreed rate (e.g. the employee's average hourly rate) for these breaks. However, employers have no obligation to pay employees a protected rate if the only job they can do is less well paid than before.

A nurse becomes disabled after a back injury. After talking to her and taking specialist advice, the employer decides that there are no reasonable adjustments that could be made to her present role. The employer then considers whether there is another role that would be suitable, and offers an alternative post to the employee, at roughly the same level of seniority. However, if after considering these steps, it is apparent that there is no alternative position on a similar salary and with similar conditions, a position on a lower salary or with worse conditions could be offered as a reasonable adjustment.[21]

It would then be for the disabled person to decide whether to accept the less well-paid job.

If a case ends up in a tribunal, it will be important for the employer to have kept records of attempts to explore reasonable adjustments, even if they have been unsuccessful. Employees are expected to act reasonably in cooperation with the employer. If attempts have been made to accommodate the worker, but have failed because of the worker's unreasonable refusal to take advantage of them, the employer's duty is discharged.

Where the tribunal finds that an employer has failed to make a reasonable adjustment the employer will be liable, because such a failure cannot be justified.

There is no qualifying period of employment necessary to make a claim to an employment tribunal for disability discrimination, and no upper limit on the amount of compensation. Damages can be given for injury to feelings as well as financial loss.

DISABILITY DISCRIMINATION ACT 2005

The Disability Discrimination Act 2005 imposes a positive duty on public authorities to promote equality of opportunity for disabled people. *A Code of Practice: the Duty to Promote Disability Equality* was published in 2005 by the Disability Rights Commission. The duty is aimed at tackling systemic, institutionalised discrimination against disabled people. Rather than providing restitution when a disabled person has been the subject of discriminatory treatment, the duty requires the public authority to be proactive in removing practices, policies and procedures that impede the full participation of disabled people in employment and public life. Public authorities include the civil service, local authorities, NHS trusts, the police, and universities and colleges.

The following example is given in the Code:

> A local authority may have a policy in place on the provision of reasonable adjustments in relation to employees and prospective employees. It may provide such adjustments when required in an individual case, but may not have systematically reviewed all person specifications and job descriptions to ensure that there is nothing in them which may deter disabled applicants from applying for employment, such as the requirement for 'stamina' in administrative posts. . . . The authority is likely to be failing in its duty to promote equality of opportunity if it continues to have such a requirement in person specifications where it is not an essential element of the job.

A breach of these provisions is not enforceable through employment tribunals, but by means of a claim to the High Court for judicial review – an expensive and complicated procedure which is unlikely to be available to the ordinary citizen unless supported by the Disability Rights Commission or a disability organisation.

Each public authority must publish a Disability Equality Scheme showing how it intends to carry out its duties. Disabled people should be involved in the development of the scheme, which should set out the steps that the authority proposes to take in fulfilment of its duty. If 3 years after publication of the scheme the authority has not done what it promised, the Disability Rights Commission can issue a compliance notice and ultimately can seek a compliance order from a county court in England and Wales or from a sheriff court in Scotland. An important aspect of the scheme should be the collecting of data. The following example is given in the Code:

> A public authority becomes aware as a result of gathering evidence by impairment type that whilst it employs a relatively high percentage of disabled people, none of its employees are people with learning difficulties. As a result, the public authority develops a recruitment strategy targeting people with learning disabilities, to ensure greater representation amongst the workforce.

ENDNOTES

1 The standard is of a 'responsible, reasonable and respectable' practitioner. *Bolitho v City and Hackney HA* [1998] AC 232.
2 Formerly the Council for the Regulation of Healthcare Professions.
3 *Kapfunde v Abbey National* [1998] IRLR 583.
4 Social Security (Administration) Act 1992.

5 Health and Safety Executive. *Management Standards for Tackling Workplace Stress.* London: Health and Safety Executive; 2004.

6 *Sutherland v Hatton* [2002] IRLR 293.

7 *Barber v Somerset County Council* [2004] IRLR 651.

8 *Hartman v South Essex Community Care and Mental Health NHS Trust* [2005] IRLR 293.

9 *Dugmore v Swansea NHS Trust* [2003] IRLR 164.

10 *Briscoe v Lubrizol Ltd* [2002] IRLR 607.

11 *Scottish Courage Ltd v Guthrie* [2004] UKEAT/0788/03.

12 *Scottish Water v McGowan* [2005] IRLR 167.

13 *East Lindsey District Council v Daubney* [1977] ICR 566.

14 *Wilson v Post Office* [2000] IRLR 834.

15 *Jones v Post Office* [2001] IRLR 384.

16 *Archibald v Fife Council* [2004] IRLR 651.

17 *Smith v Churchills Stairlifts plc* [2006] IRLR 41.

18 *Meikle v Nottinghamshire County Council* [2004] IRLR 703.

19 *O'Hanlon v Commissioners for Inland Revenue and Customs. The Times,* 13 April 2007.

20 *Callagan v Glasgow City Council* [2001] IRLR 724.

21 Disability Rights Commission. *Code of Practice: employment and occupation.* London: Disability Rights Commission; 2004.

Appendix

DOS AND DON'TS OF REHABILITATION FOR WORK FOR HEALTH PROFESSIONALS

Are your patients off sick with depression/stress?

Do:
- Treat your patient as an individual.
- Cultivate an empowering consultation style. Be:
  - friendly/accessible
  - supportive/encouraging
  - empathetic/listening
  - caring/personal.
- Make joint decisions whenever possible with regard to:
  - medication
  - sick leave
  - return to work.
- When the patient is unable to cope:
  - take over decision making temporarily
  - give back control to the patient as soon as possible.
- Offer antidepressant medication when clinically indicated to patients who want it to alleviate symptoms as a temporary crutch.
- Offer practical help/suggestions by adopting a problem-solving approach:
  - elicit, clarify and prioritise problems
  - consider the alternatives
  - identify the resources necessary.
- Offer illness management/symptom relief.
- Offer specialist referral if indicated:

- mental health
- occupational health
- counselling
- physical and psychological therapies
- social and financial advice (Citizens Advice Bureau, Jobcentre Plus).

❭ Encourage patients to:
- mobilise their own coping resources
- keep active/busy
- work out their own solutions.

❭ Give the patient/their employer a clear idea of:
- what is causing their symptoms
- how long they are likely to be off sick (if possible).

❭ Consider the relationship between illness and work.
- Find out what work involves – ask for a job description.
- Find out whether work is affecting the patient's symptoms (if it is, this suggests problems/stress at work; if it isn't, work may be providing a distraction/escape from problems at home).
- Find out whether the illness is affecting work. Consider the patient's capability/suitability for certain types of tasks. Carry out a risk assessment. Is specialist referral necessary to answer these questions?

❭ Communicate with the employer.
- Make recommendations on the patient's sick note.
- Write (as appropriate, by agreement with the patient) to the line manager human resources department, occupational health service or the patient's GP.

❭ Draw up a back-to-work plan.
- When is the patient going to be ready to return to work?
- When will staying at home make them worse rather than better?
- What limitations does the patient currently have?
- Consider recommending 'reasonable adjustments' in their workplace to facilitate job retention. These could include adjustments to hours of work (part time, phased return), changes to job/role (unfit for specified tasks), changes to the environment, or adjustments to their place of work.
- Should the decision regarding (relative) fitness for work be made by a specialist?

Don't:

) Be dismissive (e.g. by saying 'pull yourself together').

) Catastrophise (e.g. by saying 'you won't be able to do anything' or 'you're so ill').

) Pathologise symptoms of stress.

) Regard sickness certification as a 'quickie' and not requiring thought.

) Forget that the patient's employer will read the sick note (don't choose a label which may cause harm or prejudice).

) Refer the patient straight on to someone else to avoid dealing with the problem.

) Stick to guidelines and protocols which may not suit the individual.

) Encourage dependency on medication or other forms of help.

) Bully the patient into agreeing to actions or treatments that they don't want (if they don't want them they won't comply with them, so they won't benefit from them).

) Give confusing messages to the employer.

) Sign the patient off sick for long periods without review.

) Certify the patient fit for work without understanding their job requirements.

) Suggest specific workplace adjustments without understanding the patient's job requirements.

) Forget that you and your patient are human beings.

Index